Social Action with Children and Families

Me...
is n...
serv...
com...
Chi...
toge...
dev...
and...

Foc...
on...
Fan...
prof...
com...
on t...
to p...
the...
and...
with...

The...
find...

Cre...
Cult...

The State of Welfare
Edited by Mary Langan

Nearly half a century after its post-war consolidation, the British welfare state is once again at the centre of political controversy. After a decade in which the role of the state in the provision of welfare was steadily reduced in favour of the private, voluntary and informal sectors, with relatively little public debate or resistance, the further extension of the new mixed economy of welfare in the spheres of health and education became a major political issue in the early 1990s. At the same time the impact of deepening recession has begun to expose some of the deficiencies of market forces in areas, such as housing and income maintenance, where their role had expanded dramatically during the 1980s. *The State of Welfare* provides a forum for continuing the debate about the services we need in the 1990s.

Titles of related interest also in *The State of Welfare* series

The Dynamics of British Health Policy
Stephen Harrison, David Hunter and Christopher Pollitt

Radical Social Work Today
Edited by Mary Langan and Phil Lee

Taking Child Abuse Seriously
The Violence Against Children Study Group

Ideologies of Welfare: From Dreams to Disillusion
John Clarke, Allan Cochrane and Carol Smart

Women, Oppression and Social Work
Edited by Mary Langan and Lesley Day

Managing Poverty: The Limits of Social Assistance
Carol Walker

The Eclipse of Council Housing
Ian Cole and Robert Furbey

Towards a Post-Fordist Welfare State
Roger Burrows and Brian Loader

Working with Men: Feminism and Social Work
Edited by Kate Cavanagh and Viviene E. Cree

Social Theory, Social Change and Social Work
Edited by Nigel Parton

Working for Equality in Health
Edited by Paul Bywaters and Eileen McLeod

Social Action with Children and Families

A community development approach to child and family welfare

Edited by Crescy Cannan and Chris Warren

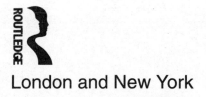

London and New York

First published 1997
by Routledge
11 New Fetter Lane, London EC4P 4EE

Simultaneously published in the USA and Canada
by Routledge
29 West 35th Street, New York, NY 10001

Typeset in Times by
Ponting–Green Publishing Services, Chesham, Bucks
Printed and bound in Great Britain by
Redwood Books, Trowbridge, Wiltshire

British Library Cataloguing in Publication Data
A catalogue record for this book is available from the
British Library

Library of Congress Cataloging in Publication Data
Social Action with Children and Families: A community
    development approach to child and family welfare / edited by
    Cressy Cannan and Chris Warren.
    (The State of Welfare)
        Includes bibliographical references and index.
        1. Social work with children.   2. Family social work.
    3. Child welfare.   I. Cannan, Cressy.   II. Warren, Chris.
    III. Series.
    HV713.S615   1996
    362.7–dc20   96–7490

ISBN   0–415–13150–2 (hbk)
ISBN   0–415–13151–0 (pbk)

Contents

Contributors

Marie-Renée Bourget-Daitch is Director of the Mouvement pour le Développement Social, a French organisation which promotes social development. She has worked in MDSL-Formation, which works on the ground with practitioners and local inhabitants to promote their participation in social development projects.

Crescy Cannan is a senior lecturer in social policy at the University of Sussex. She has a long-standing interest in French and German social welfare policy, and has built on her research on family centres to look at innovative community development approaches to promoting children's and young people's participation in society.

Jenny Clifton is a lecturer in social work at the University of Sussex. Her background is in social work and voluntary community action. Her involvement with children's rights started with the awareness that a lack of respect for children impoverishes the whole community – and a strong memory of adults who wouldn't listen.

Peter Durrant qualified as a social worker in his early thirties via a second-chance college course. Disappointed by mainstream social work's search for a professional identity and its bureaucracy, he moved into community social work. He is Co-ordinator of BASW's Special Interest Group on Community Social Work.

Annemarie Gerzer-Sass was born in 1948, and is married with two children. She is Senior Researcher at the Deutsches Jugendinstitut (German Youth Institute) in Munich, working in the field of family policy. She has a particular interest in social innovation in the welfare state.

Paul Henderson is Director of Practice Development at the Community Development Foundation. It was as a result of observing approaches to working with children in France that he started to explore the links between children and community development. He recently edited *Children and Communities* (CDF/The Children's Society, 1995).

David Hodgson, who is interested in collective action involving young people, led an initiative at the National Children's Bureau on children's participation in social work decisions before joining the National Council of Voluntary Child Care Organisations as Children's Rights Development Officer. He now lectures in social work at Kingston University.

Barry Hulyer has never been published before. Unemployable for many years, he started in community work in 1977. He was trained at Goldsmiths College, worked at a community resource centre and is now the manager of a neighbourhood community development project in Sussex.

Eva Lloyd held the policy and research brief for six years for Save the Children's work with young children and their families in the UK. Prior to that she researched day care and other early years services at London University's Thomas Coram Research Unit where she contributed to a number of publications. She now works for Barnardo's as Principal Officer, Research and Development.

Rudolph Pettinger was born in 1939, and is married with three children. He is Head of the Department of Family Research and Family Policy at the Deutsches Jugendinstitut (German Youth Institute) in Munich – a leading research centre in this field.

Jo Tunnard's interest in community development started with her work as a teacher in the north of England, followed by two years in Central America. Welfare rights work at Child Poverty Action Group was followed by thirteen years as Director of the Family Rights Group. She now works freelance and has a particular interest in family support, and the participation of users in the design, delivery and evaluation of services.

Chris Warren is a social worker and lecturer in social policy and social work at the University of Sussex. His particular interest is in community and social development as a basis for family support practice and the role of family centres in community development. He has recently completed an evaluation of the Department of Health Family Support Initiative.

Series editor's preface

In the 1990s the perception of a crisis of welfare systems has become universal across the Western world. The coincidence of global economic slump and the ending of the Cold War has intensified pressures to reduce welfare spending at the same time that Western governments, traditional social institutions and political parties all face unprecedented problems of legitimacy. Given the importance of welfare policies in securing popular consent for existing regimes and in maintaining social stability, welfare budgets have in general proved remarkably resilient even in the face of governments proclaiming the principles of austerity and self-reliance.

Yet the crisis of welfare has led to measures of reform and retrenchment which have provoked often bitter controversy in virtually every sphere, from hospitals and schools to social security benefits and personal social services. What is striking is the crumbling of the old structures and policies before any clear alternative has emerged. The general impression is one of exhaustion and confusion. There is a widespread sense that everything has been tried and has failed and that nobody is very clear about how to advance into an increasingly bleak future.

On both sides of the Atlantic, the agenda of free market anti-statism has provided the cutting edge for measures of privatisation. The result has been a substantial shift in the 'mixed economy' of welfare towards a more market-orientated approach. But it has not taken long for the defects of the market as a mechanism for social regulation to become apparent. Yet now that the inadequacy of the market in providing equitable or even efficient welfare services is exposed, where else is there to turn?

The State of Welfare series aims to provide a critical assessment of the policy implications of some of the wide social and economic changes of the 1990s. Globalisation, the emergence of post-industrial society, the transformation of work, demographic shifts and changes in gender roles and family structures all have major consequences for the patterns of welfare provision established half a century ago.

The demands of women and minority ethnic groups, as well as the voices of younger, older and disabled people and the influences of social movements concerned with issues of sexuality, gender and the environment must all be taken into account in the construction of a social policy for the new millennium.

Mary Langan
March 1995

Acknowledgements

This book grew out of the editors' shared interest in family centres, community development, and French approaches to family support. We would particularly like to thank Jean-Louis Cardi, Patricia Frin and Jean-Marie Gourvil, and their colleagues in France, for the time and help they have given us over several years.

Many other people have helped us in the development of the ideas that led to this book. They are too numerous to mention, but we hope they are pleased with the result. There are others who have helped with particular section of the book. Andrea Hammel and Christien Doyle worked on the translations. Many young people contributed to Jenny Clifton and David Hodgson's chapter, especially the ROC Festival people, VOYCE, Hove Schools' Councillors, Kate and Helen. David Hodgson would like to thank all the people with whom he worked at NCVO.

We would like to thank the following publishers for granting permission to quote material: Calouste Gulbenkian Foundation for permission to use extracts from *One Scandal too Many*; Crown copyright is reproduced with the permission of the Controller of HMSO to quote from *Family Support and Prevention: Studies in Local Areas*, edited by Jane Gibbons; Kluwer Academic Press for permission to quote extracts from Jenny Clifton and David Hodgson's chapter in *The Ideologies of Children's Rights*, edited by M. Freeman and P. Veerman; Macmillan Press Ltd for permission to quote from *Community Work*, edited by Alan Twelvetrees; Oxford University Press for permission to quote extracts from *Children's Rights and the Law*, edited by P. Alston, S. Parker, J. Seymour, chapter by John Eekelaar; Pluto Press for permission to reproduce an extract from *Children and Communities* edited by Paul Henderson; Prentice Hall for permission to use an extract from *Changing Families, Changing Welfare*, published by Harvester Wheatsheaf; Save the Children for permission to use extracts from *Childcare in the*

Community; Sweet & Maxwell for permission to quote extracts from *Journal of Social Welfare and Family Law*; Vintage/Commission on Social Justice, *Social Justice: Strategies for National Renewal.*

Introduction

Crescy Cannan and Chris Warren

We argue in this book that meeting the needs of children at the same time as promoting family life is more than a question of resources: it needs a cultural change in social services, a rediscovery and a modernisation of the social action and community development traditions in social work. We need to find ways of working together to promote environments in which children can flourish and to develop forms of public life that are friendly to children, young people and their parents.

Recent changes (both positive and negative) in child care systems have undoubtedly put more pressures on those working in them. Social workers, in whatever setting, are more open to public scrutiny and are expected to take much more account of their clients' views than in the past. They are expected to deal with or to make provision for problems arising from wide areas of their clients' or service users' lives. They are expected to work in partnership with parents and with other professionals, and with community groups.

Much of this, especially given the underfunding of the welfare state in Britain, is imposing a sense of uncertainty in social work. A central aim of this book is to help those working in this field to find a new, more positive sense of direction and purpose.We argue that children's and family services need recasting in a community development framework which we term social action, and that social workers need to draw on this strand of their profession (which has been muted over the last fifteen years) in order to share in the task of promoting child and family well-being. As the Commission on Social Justice argued in its *Strategies for National Renewal* (1994), we need to invest in our social capital, within a framework of reciprocal responsibilities between state and society:

Social capital consists of the institutions and relationships of a thriving civil society – from networks of neighbours to extended families, community groups to religious organisations, local businesses to local public services, youth clubs to parent–teacher associations, playgroups to police on the beat. Where you live, who else lives there, and how they live their lives – co-operatively or selfishly, responsibly or destructively – can be as important as personal resources in determining life chances.

(Commission on Social Justice 1994: 307–8)

This book sets out to provide accounts of how this is being done in the fields of children and family support and how empowering and participative practice can be developed and sustained.

CHILDREN'S POLICIES: THE HISTORICAL BACKGROUND

Irrespective of governments' politics, there is an apparent convergence in recent trends in social policy, in attitudes to children and to social provision for families. Most north-western European countries have newish legislation emphasising the rights of the child – to family life and to remain with his or her family where possible, to protection from abuse, and to voice an opinion over his or her circumstances and plans. Such children's legislation was passed in 1982 in Sweden, 1984 in France, 1989 in England and Wales and 1990 in Germany (Colla-Müller 1993: 87–8; Madge 1994a: 39–47).There was equivalent legislation in the USA in 1980. There is a philosophy of partnership between state and parents in helping parents meet their responsibilities, and in enabling them as far as possible to retain those responsibilities.

Such national legislation complements the UN Convention on the Rights of the Child of 1989 which stresses the rights of children to be actively involved in both the public and private spheres over matters that concern them, and asserts the family as the rightful place of abode. This stress on the family contrasts with the more libertarian approaches to children's rights of the 1960s – which sometimes stressed the repressive aspects of the family and argued for alternative modes of communal living for children's liberation (see Jenny Clifton and David Hodgson's chapter in this book for an account of views on children's rights). But circumstances in the 1990s are different. Children living independently of families are not free, but rather condemned to the risks of the street, of crime, homelessness and sexual exploitation. Views of family policy have also evolved, partly through the processes of European integration and in response to changes in family structures. Divorce, lone-parent families and never-married parents have dramatically altered the map of family life in all classes.

Part of the reason for the current precariousness of family life may be cultural, but this is outweighed by the impact of restructured labour markets upon patterns of employment both over lifetimes and between men and women. 'Flexible' labour markets mean more labour mobility, weakened communities and more temporary and part-time employment. They mean more long-term unemployment, especially among young people, thus lengthening the period of dependence of youth, whether as students or unemployed, on families and the state. It is clear then that if rising expectations of families' care of their children are to be met then families need support from the state in order to meet these responsibilities. Here there are differences between states: during the 1980s the UK took a minimalist position, arguing that the family and its responsibilities were entirely private matters except for cases of gross failure. France, at the other extreme, extended its family support, recognising the necessity of providing high-quality services to children and also promoting women as workers *and* as mothers, in short, supporting families whatever their form (Hantrais 1994: 224).

Across the European Union (EU) the use of residential children's homes is declining (Colton and Hellinckx 1994). Usually built in the late nineteenth century or early twentieth century, they were solidly bounded institutions where dangerous or damaged children spent their childhoods, quite removed from their families. Children's homes were usually run by religious or charitable associations or under the poor laws, and despite a small number of humanitarian or enlightened reformers (for instance in settlements, youth organisations, and some progressive education movements), they overwhelmingly contained rather than developed their children. Horizons were low, with inmates usually prepared for manual work in domestic or military service or in agricultural labouring.

Although there was some development of community services in the first half of this century, real change began in Britain with the 1948 Children Act. Social workers (then called child care or children's officers) provided family-based help for 'problem families' from local authority Children's Departments. These state services were never intended for the majority of children or families, but were rather a residual service for those who had failed to 'manage' their family lives through the universal services – education and health – and through social housing. Alongside these state services were voluntary organisations such as the Family Service Units, whose workers, originally conscientious objectors in the second world war, worked intensively with 'problem families' in a spirit of practical help and solidarity.

These approaches, although criticised in the 1960s as variously patronising or ineffectual, nevertheless began to create welfare services for families in which boundaries were lowered, children went in *and out* of (and maybe back into) care; many poor families relied on children's homes, foster parents and day nurseries to tide them over their crises. Services began to be more flexible, with a landmark in the 1963 Children and Young Persons Act. This explicitly stressed a preventive outlook, and enabled authorities to spend money to keep children with their families, for instance by paying for playgroup places, family aides, holiday schemes, home improvements and so forth.

The 'Seebohm' social services departments, created in 1971, integrated welfare services and social workers in the fields of child care, mental welfare, disability and old age into a generic, community-based system. Personal social services were now to be provided in such a way that they enhanced local networks and communities, and social services departments became major employers of community workers until the later 1970s. This community development strand of social work was invigorated by the Community Development Projects established in the late 1960s, bringing some of the imagination of the US War on Poverty programmes. The rediscovery of poverty in the 1960s and the emergence of articulate pressure groups such as the Child Poverty Action Group also fuelled radical community movements and those within social work – which was suddenly rejuvenated by the expansion of the social sciences in the then new universities. These movements argued for rights – of psychiatric patients, prisoners, school children, black people and families dissatisfied with the social services. The state was understood as an agent of social control of the working class and social workers should ensure that they worked for their clients and communities and not the state.

It was the women's movement that moved this left-libertarianism into a position more akin to that of today. Feminists argued that an undifferentiated notion of family or parental rights obscured the different interests and power balances within families. The radical left debate then shifted from a critique of the state's agents to debating ways in which social workers and other professionals could work with their clients to counter various forms of oppression, and especially sexism and racism, at a personal as well as a political level. Oppression is no longer seen as resting simplistically in the state but as embedded in all the public and private institutions of society, which simultaneously contain opportunities and discrimination.

The radical right however, which came to power in the UK in 1979, built on earlier criticisms of professionals and notably on media attacks on cases where social workers' intervention in families suspected of child abuse had been destructive of those families (for example, Campbell 1988). The neo-conservative project became a programme of restructuring the welfare state by apparently empowering consumers and new cadres of managers, and thus constraining welfare state professionals' autonomy. These forces, combined with the further residualisation of welfare services in the UK and the USA, twisted social services departments' views of what family and children's services should be like. During the 1980s it seemed as if the only area of growth in social services (including the voluntary sector) was in projects centring on the treatment or prevention of child abuse. Social workers found that they were, in the main, dealing only with the most severe cases of need or danger.

CONTEMPORARY CHILDREN'S POLICIES: CHILDREN'S RIGHTS AND PARENTS' RESPONSIBILITIES

The emphasis on child abuse is clearly no way for social services departments to tackle today's massive problems of family need and child and youth disadvantage, and there are signs of change. The Children Act of 1989 reflected concerns about the overuse of judicial mechanisms in child care work. It stressed negotiation and the duty of local authorities to safeguard the welfare of children in need as far as possible within their family homes, and, in Part 3, Schedule 2, provides the legislative framework for family support. Subsequently, two government publications, the Audit Commission report, *Seen but not Heard* (1994), and a Department of Health review of research findings on child protection (DoH 1995) expressed concern about the continuing emphasis on child protection enquiry in the work of social services departments. So there has been something of a re-think at official levels. The emerging focus on promoting children's rights and parents' responsibilities is, as we have seen, consistent with trends in other European countries and in North America.

How should these ideas be put into practice? While ideas of family support have grown, the use of residential institutions has shrunk, and changed. Quality residential (or day) care is expensive, especially if modern ideas on health, education and personal development, such as those enshrined in the UN Convention, are to be met. Over the last twenty years there has been a consensus that smaller-scale units are more conducive (whether for children or for people with disabilities or mental health problems) to developing and helping rather than containing their residents and users (Colton and Hellinckx 1994). Across north-western Europe there has been a fall in the numbers of children and young people in residential care (for instance a fall of about one-third in France and Belgium since 1979 (Madge 1994a: 50–1) and increasing use of foster care. To some extent this movement followed from evidence that children who grew up in care were at risk of becoming homeless, having psychiatric problems, entering prisons, becoming young unsupported parents and so forth (the evidence is reviewed in Madge (1994b) and Colton and Hellinckx (1993, 1994)).

Children's homes have become much more diverse, flexible settings, partly to contain costs but also as new settings of family support. The best – and this includes former children's homes which have become family centres – combine day and residential provision, welcoming and involving parents, offering different kinds of specialist provision, acting as resource centres for families in need or for child minders and foster parents. Residents (young or old, of whatever abilities, and their workers) no longer spend all aspects of their lives in the total institution. Instead they 'normalise' their lives using schools, leisure and health services with other citizens, and wherever possible integrating their lives with their own families, even if in public care (Colton *et al.* 1991; Madge 1994a).

There are spectrums of provision, including foyers for teenagers and young workers (particularly in France). In Germany there is a range of types of unit, from unsupported shared flats to small staffed communes which draw on a range of support, for instance from social pedagogues (children and youth workers) based in local programmes for young people (Colla-Müller 1993: 80–2). In most countries there are now intensive, community-based and residential therapeutic schemes for victims of sexual abuse. So, the boundaries have become more flexible between residential and day institutions, between being in public care and being the responsibility of parents, or, for older children and young people, being cared for and being independent. There is a recognition in France, Flanders, the Netherlands, Germany and Sweden that general services and benefits need to be improved to enable parents to look after their children adequately, and that many kinds of families will need or should be encouraged to use various kinds of day centres and after-school centres, or to receive more intensive help. This help should not substitute for their parenting but assist it, and rather than being targeted only on the most desperate, it should integrate people with each other, bringing

different types of people together with different strengths, to promote
networks and solidarity.

This is of course the spirit of the English and Welsh 1989 Children
Act in that it removes the status of being 'in care' (and thus beyond
parental responsibility) and introduces the notion of 'children in need'
for whom local authorities are empowered to provide a range of services
to promote them and their families. This is an important difference from
the earlier, narrower notion of 'preventing reception into care', which
offered first aid to families but did little to promote their capacities and
resources. Family centres, recognised in the Act (Schedule 2/9), have
emerged as a key mechanism of supporting families by helping them
promote their children's welfare (Warren 1993). As we shall see, there
are significant differences between those which treat referred families in
the old manner and those which support a wide range of families and
local people in the framework of community development. It is to these
we now turn.

NEIGHBOURHOOD FAMILY CENTRES: A NEW
PARADIGM IN WELFARE STATES

It is possible to see the development of family centres – from the late 1970s
– as a barometer of social and community work within a changing welfare
state. To some extent family centres have emerged from growing pluralism
and thus the changing role of the voluntary sector. Major voluntary
organisations like The Children's Society had found their market in
residential provision declining and sought to provide new services. At the
same time social services departments were looking for ways to deal with
the increasing needs of children, and particularly abuse within the family.
Such changes coincided with a recognition of systems and whole-family
thinking in social work and family centres were born. The Family Rights
Group was set up in the same period in opposition to the fierce ideologies
of 'child rescue' in adoption and fostering departments in the immediate
post-1975 Act era, again pushing social services departments towards
better ways of working with families than tended to be found in the area
social services team. Family centres – which have proved to be a dynamic
innovation in welfare practice – are still evolving in interesting ways.

Adamson and Warren (1983), describing family centres of the early
1980s, identified what was essentially an adapted day care facility, a kind
of resource centre, which had the following features:

• an emphasis on neighbourhood;
• the capacity to engage families through a unique combination of
  building, play facilities, meeting space, range of activities from the

very practical, including food, to a group of relatively sophisticated interventions like family therapy and intensive counselling;

• continuity and containment through the regularity of agreements about attending and the ability of the centre team to embrace the variety of issues which families face;
• a flexibility of approach and staff background;
• a stress on participation, through user groups, open records, consultative groups of various kinds, or through the use of volunteers;
• a resource centre to the local community;
• above all there is, or is said to be, a focus on the whole family, and services are orientated as much towards parents as they are towards children.

By the end of the 1980s Warren (1991) had enumerated 353 family centres in a survey of family centres in local authorities and voluntary organisations in England and Wales and by that time local authorities' social services departments had become the main providers of family centres. The indications were that local authority family centres (and voluntary sector centres with service agreements with local authorities) were distinguished from the more promotional styles of many of the voluntary sector centres by an emphasis on referral from area teams and assessment as part of child protection procedures. Family centres thus mirrored late 1970s and 1980s child and family social policy.

Since then evidence has accumulated showing that family support services operate most effectively (according to users as well as professionals) from centres that are open to their local neighbourhood and have a diversity of activities for a wide range of users (Cannan 1992; Gibbons et al. 1990; Gibbons 1992; Holman 1988; Smith 1993). These neighbourhood-oriented family centres are a recent success story (the literature is reviewed by Eva Lloyd in her chapter in this book). Evidence, which comes from the UK and the USA and from France and Germany, shows that these centres reach large numbers of people, and encourage user ownership of the centre, thus reducing stigma, and raising users' self-esteem and confidence. They also contribute to local friendship networks and enable parents to participate in their local community and in their children's social worlds. They have enabled many parents to make the transition from helped to voluntary or paid helper, and to gain training, education and employment.

(Family support services from neighbourhood centres then have a particular quality which cannot be replicated in the bureaucratic offices of social services departments.)Users like the rounded approach to their needs.(There are activities for children as well as parents. There are counselling and therapeutic services as well as leisure and educational activities. There is a focus on individual users as well as their local neighbourhood. Many family centres bridge the generations, with activities for all ages of children, for youth and elderly people as well as parents)

This genericism connects with the holistic approach that is increasingly argued for by those promoting the welfare and rights of children. (Childhood has many facets – psychological, educational, social, health and so it needs an integrated social response. This is especially so when considering children in need: poverty is multi-dimensional and parents need help on many levels to overcome its effects – counselling, credit unions, health advice, training and adult education, leisure activities and environmental improvements)(Henderson 1995). Caring too is a holistic activity demanding rounded, long-term rather than sectorised support services. Centre-based services, especially those which enable parents to use their own energies and build friendship networks have been increasingly used in Germany as a better matched public response to parent support than the fragmented, task-oriented social services office (see Annemarie Gerzer-Sass and Rudolph Pettinger in this book).

(It is amongst the voluntary organisations that we see the greatest expression of practice akin to empowerment practice. At best, centre practitioners hold values and also provide opportunities that reflect the empowerment journey. There is an emphasis on an open and protective environment for parent and child, a focus on women as oppressed people, disentangling the problems and setting shared tasks, a combination of interpersonal, educational and practical help, a journey from individual help, counselling and peer-group support, to the creation of education and work opportunities for women)

Such practices, though stressing the containing and expressive side of social intervention, are nevertheless closely tied to community development principles by which, through individual and collective action, people identify their own potential, understand the processes of internalisation of oppression which disable them, and participate in the mainstream rather than the margins of communities. In small ways so far, family centres have sought to link the local and the global. Some individual centres have worked hard at making alliances between users, not only regionally but internationally.

This distinction between the promotional styles of the voluntary sector centres and the assessment and protection styles of the local authority centres is not necessarily helpful. It stereotypes approaches in ways which ignore the political and financial constraints and the statutory duties upon local authorities. It also ignores the evidence of good practice where it is to be found in local authorities, some of whom, by working in partnerships between social services, health, education and a range of voluntary and community groups, have created successful and popular centres that can operate at both protection and community development levels. (An example is the Penn Green centre in Corby (Audit Commission 1994).) Some voluntary organisations simply contract to provide assessment and child protection services with the social services department; promotional and empowering work is not, then, synonymous with the voluntary sector, though it has been largely associated with it. The way ahead lies not in the separation of these two but through multi-agency partnerships which include user groups and local associations. In this way the statutory or voluntary distinction could become outmoded, though unfortunately public expenditure restrictions make the development of local integrated strategies for families, children and youth a precarious business.

Centres then, for all their problems of context and experience of families' disasters, are also full of stories of extraordinary journeys from hopelessness to autonomy. Their workers can claim to be empowerment practitioners though operating at the beginning stage of the empowerment journey (an idea developed by Chris Warren in his chapter in this book). What they might fairly complain of is that they are the only provision in the local service network so that people's possibilities of change are limited. Our argument, which will be sustained by the contributions in this book, is that family centre practice as a whole offers a new paradigm for practice. It is still beset by pathological assumptions, of blaming, of patterns of rescue, but offers nevertheless a model and a setting for integrated family support practice in the context of child-focused provision.

NEW SOCIAL ACTION AND THE CHANGING WELFARE STATES OF EUROPE

Mainstream social work has, under pressure, too easily turned its back on the social action of new social movements (for instance of people with disabilities) and of the independent welfare organisations and found a sense of purpose in clinical approaches and in the detailing of assessment and treatment procedures for children victimised in their families. Family centres have too often become settings for this narrow kind of practice, and conversely the workers in the community-oriented centres of voluntary agencies are often hostile to social services and do not consider themselves to be social workers. Yet many family centres and community projects have, as we have seen, kept alive imaginative ways of working with families and children alongside developing their communities. It is to some of these new forms of social action that we now turn, having argued that family centres are developing a new paradigm of intervention. What lessons are there in the wider, changing field of social welfare?

Paradoxically, the new right British government, hostile to the welfare state, has, in its enterprise policies and in breaking the state monopoly in health and community care, expanded opportunities for community work (Mayo 1994). At the same time, local authorities, especially those in large cities with Labour councils, have, since the early 1980s, been recasting their role not merely as enablers but as strategic planners. Here we find the rhetoric, as in EU anti-poverty and urban development programmes, of partnership, participation and integrated approaches in socio-economic regeneration (e.g. Commission of the EC 1992). Government intitiatives of the 1990s such as City Challenge or the Single Regeneration Budget have used some of the same language in pursuing the goals of economic regeneration, alongside attempts such as Safer Cities, to control the slide into crime and violence that unemployment has brought to the poorer areas of cities. Critics remark, though, that they fail to place sufficient emphasis on 'the need to build linkages between the economic, human and social capital investments required to achieve sustainable regeneration' (Commission on Social Justice 1994: 325), or to link the 'soft' issues of local people's needs and experience with the 'hard' issues of economic regeneration (see Paul Henderson's chapter in this book).

The increasingly strategic approach in socio-economic planning alongside a restructuring of health and social services is not, then, only a right-wing phenomenon. Across north-western Europe we find user groups and new social movements challenging professionals' authority. In the community care field this is especially so of people with disabilities, learning difficulties and mental illness, and of their carers. Consumers are demanding a greater voice. Classic Beveridge-style post-war welfare states (of whatever model) are becoming outmoded because they impose a passivity on people who require services; needs and services are determined by experts, and the unemployed are marginalised from useful life. This discourse was developed by the right in the UK in the 1980s and by the socialists in France at the same time (see Crescy Cannan's chapter in this book). States have come up with various strategies for combating the exclusion of unemployment, but all emphasise in some form opportunities, even responsibilities, to participate in society. It seems unlikely that full employment will return, so new forms of social participation, of solidarity, need to be devised if society is not to fracture. These forms of participation can themselves promote welfare in ways that this book will consider.

These questions have led to a re-emergence of community development methods in the social welfare field as local authorities have modified their styles and organisation of service delivery to build more effective relationships between themselves and their consumers (McConnell 1991). There have been, for instance, the Dutch Sociale Vernieuwing programme (from 1989) and the debureaucratisation and self-help movement in Germany (Grunow 1986), which, like the French Développement Social des Quartiers programme, linked the transformation of outmoded welfare states with socio-economic regeneration and the combating of exclusion (Robbins 1994). There is an increasing linkage of promotive social welfare and community development with the idea of social development in the Third World. International aid agencies have pointed to the fact that economic growth in developing countries does not necessarily trickle down, and that prosperity can and does widen inequalities. Thus economic development requires social welfare to ensure that its benefits are shared in accordance with principles of social justice.

Social development as an idea has spread. Since the first International Conference on Social Development in Hong Kong in 1980 there has been growing interest, an appreciation that developed countries could learn from strategies in developing countries (Elliott 1993). There is a sense that the consequences of growth combined with competitive economic policies in the West and in the former communist countries are producing dangerous mixes of crime, family disintegration, long-term (youth) unemployment, nationalism and xenophobia. Social development implies a mix of values and practices: popular participation, unified socio-economic planning, advocacy, distributive justice, social education, appropriate technology, institution-building, empowerment and preventive rather than remedial and residual approaches (Midgley 1995).

The European region of the International Council on Social Welfare (1994) has also committed itself to the principles and practices of social development and called on the UN to adopt a Social Charter similar to the Council of Europe Social Charter in order that governments would have to integrate social rights and associated governmental responsibilities into national legislation. It saw the issues of participation, equal opportunities and full citizenship for all as crucial issues facing the European region with its 18 million unemployed in Western Europe and many more in east and central Europe, raising serious problems for democracy in the future (Rasmussen and Pijl 1994). The social development approach then is renewing the older community development tradition by linking social and economic policy more closely, by doing so within clearly stated principles of social justice, by focusing its efforts on those who most need empowering, and by introducing green principles of sustainability. In doing so it offers social work a new social approach and philosophy, which modernises and makes effective the community work of the 1960s.

This approach offers us the possibilities of seeing welfare imaginatively, as a decentralised *process* rather than professionally determined *service*. Welfare can be created from interrelated community, citizen and user groups who are able to work in partnership with accountable professionals and experts who adapt their approaches to meet local conditions. This requires professionals to work more closely both with community groups and with other professionals – the interagency and partnership approaches. This then is a contemporary challenge to social workers, who because of the weight of responsibilities for child abuse often find it difficult to move out of familiar bureaucratic settings to working in more open ways. Yet it is happening, with, for instance, preventive community development teams re-appearing in British social services departments. As we have seen, family centres, at their best, try to develop personal, social and economic capacities at the local level, promoting not just parenting skills, but the broader fields of opportunity, education, natural and built environment, health and networks, which underpin people's capacities to care for each other.

Another sign of change at the local level is the interest in the social economy (or social firms, social enterprise or the social market) which community projects and community care workers are developing. This interest may be a far more 'green' and sustainable one than the stress on growth and competition in EU economic policy and in both Labour and Conservative parties in the UK. Armstrong (1994) in his evaluation of EU urban regeneration projects argues that the social enterprise sector, midway between commercially viable businesses and voluntary activities, has often been overlooked in regeneration schemes though it can provide both local services and some paid employment. The social economy introduces principles of co-operation and sharing (surplus is for community benefit or reinvestment), social concern and responsibility for the economic, social and environmental problems of their area. A developed social economy – as a concrete, local twin to the global economy – could highlight the value of unpaid as well as paid work and provide a stratum of small independent and voluntary organisations which not only make life tolerable, but help people into the labour market (Cresy Cannan and Peter Durrant discuss the lessons from this sector in their chapters of this book).

From this point of view, the word 'service' is outmoded, conjuring up as it does the strong boundary between user and organisation. Instead professionals could use their expert knowledge and skills to help citizens determine these services, to plan and develop new ones and to reshape neighbourhood and city life (Marie-Renée Bourget-Daitch and Chris Warren give a French example in their chapter of this book). In east/central Europe we see new welfare initiatives emerging from the bottom up, seeing social welfare as part and parcel of the task of reconstructing civil society. We need then, learning from both the advanced welfare states of Western Europe, and the reconstructions in east/central Europe, to see social welfare as in essence the development of opportunities for inclusion, not exclusion, for participative citizenship. It seems to us that this approach is the one we need to take forward, drawing on contemporary community work, community education and neighbourhood project/family centre practices in the UK, and from the bigger social development partnerships on the continent with their stress on promoting solidarity and the social economy.

OVERVIEW OF OUR THEMES AND CHAPTERS

As we have said, we have aimed to put together a book that will provide examples of innovative contemporary social practices in the field of family support and children's well-being. The following are the themes which have emerged from our work, with an indication of how contributors have focused on them.

Children and carers need holistic and integrated rather then sectorised services. As Peter Durrant (Chapter 3) shows there are many lessons from contemporary practice in the community care field – especially in the area of adults with learning difficulties. Despite shortages in national funding, creative local strategies and even solutions are emerging. For children and their families poverty, lack of suitable public spaces, health and public safety come together to affect life chances and the quality of life. Jenny Clifton and David Hodgson (Chapter 2) show how, in working with young people to enable them to participate in matters that concern them, professionals have to question their habits of thought and divisions of labour. Working together – across agencies, sectors, professions, and in partnership with user groups and the informal sector – is emerging as a necessary strategy in social action for children and families. Paul Henderson (Chapter 1) argues that consequently community development, social, youth and community work all need to rediscover their links.

Children and parents are better helped by supporting them in their public sphere rather than by attempting to treat their private world. While there will always be a small minority of people for whom compulsory social intervention or clinical treatments are necessary, the vast majority of children in need suffer from poverty. Given that poor people tend to live in poor areas where the social infrastructure and environment are also impoverished, it is evident that any attempt to support such children must start by helping local people to shape that environment and in so doing to create opportunities for participation and a meaningful public life. Annemarie Gerzer-Sass and Rudolph Pettinger (Chapter 6) show how, in Germany, family centres have become an important focus for neighbourhoods and that they consciously try to create spaces in which all age groups can interact in a climate that is more accepting of the caring, expressive aspect of people's lives than is the modern, atomised, child-hostile and competitive world.

Further, centres can provide a space for children which is often not available to the urban child – of any class – where there is safe play and a freedom from routines and structures. In Britain, day care, after-school care and youth activities are much-needed but scarce services. Crescy Cannan (Chapter 4) looks at centres in France and shows that the provision of opportunities for children to mix, for 'socialisation', is as important a goal as the provision of day care for mothers to work or train. Both France and Germany thus provide examples of child care strategies which rest in helping children to develop the capacity for getting on with people – and which stress that learning about citizenship is as important for children as early-years education.

Family centres then can help to create communities in the round or what Barry Hulyer calls 'coherent communities'. They overcome the artificial separations of ages and other social divisions and help people integrate, make new connections and networks and solidarities as the French and Germans would say. At the same time neighbourhood-oriented family centres can help overcome the often false distinction between families referred by social services, because they have been defined as inadequate in some way, and those who are 'normal' but living in difficult circumstances. As Jenny Clifton and David Hodgson argue, from a children's rights perspective family support and child protection strategies should be reconciled. This would mean reappraising the relationship between children, families and communities.

Neighbourhood family centres epitomise a new paradigm of welfare. The old idea of departmental 'services' administered by distinct groups of professionals is no longer appropriate to the contemporary political culture or demands on the welfare state. Family centres at their best are places where local families contribute as well as receive services; the distinction between professional and service user is increasingly blurred. Flexible child care and open access to the centre are a successful formula because this is what – in France and Germany as well as Britain – parents want. It meshes with the contemporary realities of family life and employment patterns. Eva Lloyd (Chapter 7) considers the research evidence on this kind of family centre and shows how the Save the Children Fund has been able to develop highly participative centres with a strong focus on adult education (both formal and informal) which create a sense of community in areas that might have seemed beyond hope.

All this raises new questions for professionals: working alongside users, helping user groups take on some service provision, letting go of notions of how things should be done, coping with anxiety about child protection responsibilities. These issues are explored by Peter Durrant who gives some ideas from community social work and community care. Marie-Renée Bourget-Daitch and Chris Warren (Chapter 10) describe a French network of professionals (Mouvement pour le Développement Social Local – Formation) who work with local people where there are social development projects to help those local people make best use of the experts in their area so that their voices are heard in planning and strategies. Annemarie Gerzer-Sass and Rudolph Pettinger (Chapter 6) argue that it is where professionals have been able to work side by side with the 'unqualified' volunteer or parent, and where there is a genuine partnership between formal welfare providers and family self-help groups in Germany that we find the most effective child and family support.

Working with children in community development raises questions of the skills of professionals. Paul Henderson, Barry Hulyer, and Jenny Clifton and David Hodgson argue that we need to develop methods that take into account the relevant developmental stages of children, especially when helping them to participate in a rights framework. We need simultaneously to recognise children's rights to protection, autonomy and participation in spheres that concern them.

Working in partnership with parents is something which Jo Tunnard

(Chapter 8) explores in her description of the family group conference project, which was originally developed in New Zealand as a means of empowering families in their dealings with social services agencies. Families are helped to get together to consider the problem and to take collective responsibility for a plan which protects and respects the relevant children. She also considers the family advocacy project of the Family Rights Group and, like Chris Warren (Chapter 5), argues that empowerment is a process as well as a goal, something which Chris Warren calls a journey, often begun, as he shows, in family centres or the family support projects he has looked at.

This new kind of welfare strategy takes time. The majority of British family and neighbourhood projects are short term, or exist in a perpetual struggle for funding. Communities (and we leave aside questions of definition) are living things and they take time to develop; Barry Huyler gives a narrative of his own long-term community work on a particular estate, showing that a small team of workers and a centre can make a difference, even with precarious funding; stable funding of even quite modest projects could certainly achieve results as other contributors show. Paul Henderson criticises the concept of economic regeneration, arguing that it is remote from the organic needs and lives of local people: he prefers to use the term anti-exclusion – which again needs time and stability for sustainable results.

Finally, we and our contributors argue that family support and community development have to go together in a way which does not leave impoverished neighbourhoods and hard-pressed voluntary organisations to solve society's structural problems. In France and Germany there is a clear statutory responsiblity on the state to support family life and share the 'burden' of raising children; in Britain and the USA this is less clear. The recent stress on parental responsibilities is one that must be backed by top-down responsibility for helping people to parent. Bottom-up, grassroots initiatives need to be complemented by social and economic development strategies that bring resources to communities as well as the means for local professionals and activists to work together to devise locally relevant strategies. Most of all day care, after-school care and safe, imaginative environments for children need public funding, because it is on that foundation that successful families and family centres rest.

REFERENCES

Adamson, J. and Warren, C. (1983) *Welcome to St Gabriel's Family Centre!*,
    London: The Children's Society.

Armstrong, J. (1994) *Community Involvement in Urban Regeneration – a study for the European Commission (DGXVI): Interim Report (Summary)*, London: Community Development Foundation.

Audit Commission (1994) *Seen but not Heard: Coordinating Community Child Health and Social Services for Children in Need*, London: HMSO.

Campbell, B. (1988) *Unofficial Secrets: Child Sexual Abuse – the Cleveland Case*, London: Virago.

Cannan, C. (1992) *Changing Families, Changing Welfare: Family Centres and the Welfare State*, Hemel Hempstead: Harvester Wheatsheaf.

Colla-Müller, H. (1993) 'Germany', in M. J. Colton and W. Hellinckx (eds), *Child Care in the EC: A Country-Specific Guide to Foster and Residential Care*, Aldershot: Arena/Ashgate Publishing.

Colton, M. J. and Hellinckx, W. (eds) (1993) *Child Care in the EC: A Country-Specific Guide to Foster and Residential Care*, Aldershot: Arena/Ashgate Publishing.

Colton, M., and Hellinckx, W. (1994) 'Residential and foster care in the European Community: current trends in policy and practice', *British Journal of Social Work*, 24: 559–76.

Colton, M., Hellinckx, W., Bullock, R. and van den Bruel, B. (1991) 'Caring for troubled children in Flanders, the Netherlands, and the United Kingdom', *British Journal of Social Work*, 21: 381–92.

Commission of the European Communities (1992) 'Urban social development', *Social Europe*, supplement 1/92, Brussells: DGV.

Commission on Social Justice (1994) *Strategies for National Renewal*, London: Vintage.

Cox, D. (1994) 'Social development and social work education state of the art: an Asia–Pacific perspective', paper from the 1994 International Association of Schools of Social Work Congress, distributed by Manchester Metropolitan University.

DoH (Department of Health) (1995) *Child Protection: Messages from Research*, London: HMSO.

Elliott, D. (1993) 'Social work and social development: towards an integrative model for social work practice', *International Social Work*, 36: 21–36.

Gibbons, J. (ed.) (1992) *The Children Act 1989 and Family Support: Principles into Practice*, London: HMSO.

Gibbons, J., Thorpe, S. and Wilkinson, P. (1990) *Family Support and Prevention: Studies in Local Areas*, London: HMSO.

Grunow, D. (1986) 'Debureaucratisation and the self-help movement: towards a restructuring of the welfare state in the Federal Republic of Germany?', in E. Øyen (ed.), *Comparing Welfare States and their Futures*, Aldershot: Gower.

Hantrais, L. (1994) 'Family policy in Europe', in R. Page and J. Baldock (eds), *Social Policy Review 6*, Canterbury: Social Policy Association/University of Kent.

Henderson, P. (1995) 'Introduction' to P. Henderson (ed.) *Children and Communities*, London: Pluto Press/Community Development Foundation.

Holman, B. (1988) *Putting Families First: Prevention and Childcare – a Study of Prevention by Statutory and Voluntary Agencies*, Basingstoke: Macmillan.

International Council on Social Welfare (1994) 'A call for an integrated social development strategy for all', *Scandinavian Journal of Social Welfare*, 3, 4: 233–9.

McConnell, C. (1991) 'Community development in five European countries', *Community Development Journal*, 26, 2: 103–11.

Madge, N. (1994a) *Children and Residential Care in Europe*, London: European Children's Centre/National Children's Bureau.

Madge, N. (1994b) 'Extrafamilial care: short-term and long-term outcomes', in M. J. Colton *et al.* (eds), *The Art and Science of Caring: Current Research on Child Care in Europe*, Aldershot: Avebury.

Mayo, M. (1994) *Communities and Caring: The Mixed Economy of Welfare*, Basingstoke: Macmillan.

Midgley, J. (1995) *Social Development: The Developmental Perspective in Social Welfare*, London: Sage.

Rasmussen, H. C and Pijl, M. A. (eds) (1994) 'Some reflections on social development in Europe: a contribution to the UN Summit on Social Development', *Bulletin of the European Region of ICSW*.

Robbins, D. (1994) *Observatory on National Policies to Combat Social Exclusion*, Third Annual Report, Commission of the European Communities, DGV, Brussels.

Smith, T. (1993) *Six Projects run by The Children's Society: Final Report to the Department of Health and The Children's Society*, University of Oxford.

Warren, C. (1991) 'The potential for parent advocacy in family centres', unpublished M.Phil thesis, Southampton University.

Warren, C. (1993) *Family Centres and the Children Act*, Arundel: Tarrant Publications.

Part I

New strategies in social action

Chapter 1

Community development and children

A contemporary agenda

Paul Henderson

INTRODUCTION

Community development in Britain is in danger of being dominated by the demands of economists and planners. In this chapter I shall justify this statement, and go on to argue that it is an unhealthy state of affairs for community development in general and for work with children in particular.

There is an urgent need for community development to regain its confidence to articulate work on the so-called 'soft' issues of communities – community care, children, youth work – as compared with the 'hard' issues of economic development, employment and housing. The extent to which some inner-city areas, council estates and coalfield communities are experiencing increasing levels of deprivation makes this a political priority. The idea that 'comfortable' Britain can turn its back on this situation is both morally unacceptable and socially unrealistic.

It is in the most deprived areas that children suffer the worst injustices. The chapter will go on to outline ways in which community development can contribute significantly to giving them a voice. Fortunately, the danger of maintaining the false dichotomy between 'soft' and 'hard' issues is being recognised, and I conclude by making the case for integration between the two and for community development knowledge and skills to be re-assessed accordingly.

REGENERATION

In the mid-1980s, a community development project in Rochdale run by the Community Development Foundation helped to establish a community initiative among the town's Kashmiri population. Aimed at creating a focal point for young people, the initiative grew out of a youth club set up by local people. For several years it was successful in attracting local authority grants and it operated as a generalist community resource. However, from the end of the 1980s it began to rely increasingly on grants and contracts from the Department of Employment and the European Social Fund, with the result that its activities became focused on employment training. Basically, it ceased to be a community development project.

The experience of the Kashmiri Youth project (KYP) of moving from a community to a predominantly economic framework has been mirrored in many community projects throughout the country. In KYP's case it was the funding system that pushed it in that direction. In many other instances, however, the shift has been the result of the hold that the concept of regeneration has over practice and policy. If community development is now tied so closely to economics, the watchword that secures the link is 'regeneration'. For the following reasons I believe that the dominance of this concept is in danger of subverting community development.

1 *Regeneration is aligned to physical changes* – factories, offices and housing – which lead to more jobs as well as improved housing standards. Historically, regeneration is a development planners' concept, concerned above all with large-scale investment. When implemented in a crude form, as experienced in parts of London's docklands in the 1970s, it produced a reaction from community groups committed to the future of neighbourhood as opposed to the development of enterprises across much larger areas. There have been improvements since then. Yet the importance of the physical environment in regeneration means that it can be antipathetic to the small scale and to differences between communities. This, as will be seen, is inherently problematic for community development.

2 *Regeneration is overtly 'top-down'.* It works on the assumption that specified areas have 'degenerated' and expects agencies to formulate objectives and performance indicators to engineer change (sometimes literally). Community development principles of responding to felt/expressed needs and of proceeding at the pace of the community can go out of the window.

There have been instances where consultants have recommended excluding local people from consultations for fear of upsetting the plans of developers and investors. That kind of thinking shows how easy it is for community groups to be conceived as means to an end, a way of smoothing or delivering a powerful regeneration programme controlled from outside the community. Community workers should be wary when they come across phrases such as 'Local communities are key players in the regeneration process'! There is a real danger of 'community packages' being imposed, flying in the face of different experiences, needs and resources of communities.

3   *Regeneration is too narrow a concept for community development.* Policy makers have become more aware that 'effective regeneration requires attention to more than narrow economic or environmental initiatives' (Thomas 1995: 37). This is welcome. So too is the inclusion, in the bidding documents of the Single Regeneration Budget, of social as well as economic criteria.

However, community development is too important to have to fit a single framework. If community development agencies rely exclusively on a strategy of trying to broaden the agendas of regeneration agencies, they miss the point that community development can be used in a wide range of situations, and that they can do this on their terms, not always those of planners and economists. Nowhere is this more important than in work with and for children whose situation in neighbourhoods is affected by a number of forces.

4   *Regeneration falls into the trap of mystification.* It is experienced as reification, of talking in the abstract language of things rather than the language of people and objects. It is best illustrated by regeneration's use of the language of capacity building. I remain perplexed by this term because it appears to ignore the language of change and development rooted in community and adult education. It sits uneasily with community development's concern with the tangible, the importance of acting within the experiences and culture of local people. For community development to allow its links with this tradition to atrophy would be an enormous loss.

5   *Regeneration is atheoretical.* There is little evidence to date that regeneration has developed its own theory about communities and community involvement. Community development can be accused of having confusing, poorly articulated theories, but theory it does have. As a result it is possible to debate why certain actions or approaches are or are not acceptable. There is a value basis to community development which is conspicuously absent from regeneration.

If the above critique is put in the historical context of community development, the extent to which the latter now exists predominantly in an economic framework becomes doubly apparent: the origins of community development lie in the social work and education sectors. Both have influenced the development of community development practice and theory. The problem has been that both failed to develop an economic analysis of 'community'. They did not come forward with ideas for responding to the collapse of local economies. It is hardly surprising, therefore, that regeneration has claimed so much of the community development territory.

In terms of responding to the economic causes of fragmented, declining communities, the energy within the regeneration movement is obviously welcome. So too are the concerns of the government to ensure that its programmes are strongly community-based. My concern is that community development, in its eagerness to support regeneration programmes, risks losing its distinctiveness.

The case for a rigorous examination of whether or not community development is, unwittingly in most instances, acting as a handmaiden to prevailing political and economic imperatives, rests not only on an analysis of the limitations of a regeneration framework but also on an analysis of the issues and problems being experienced in Britain's most deprived areas. It is to the latter area that we now turn.

COMMUNITIES, POVERTY AND CHILDREN

The test-bed for community development lies in its capacity to respond meaningfully to the question: who gets involved, who participates? Arguably it is not that difficult to achieve citizen participation of some kind. But community development should never be understood simply as a mechanism for facilitating general notions of participation. It must always be interested in the quality of participation, particularly as this relates to issues of gender, race and class. Community development exists because it has a value-based commitment to working with the excluded of society, those people who are too poor, too oppressed or too alienated to be confident about getting involved in community activities. And to support this commitment there are tried and tested methods and skills to draw upon in the practice and evaluation of community development.

In this sense, community development must judge itself harshly. It must constantly ask the question, who are the excluded and where do they live? From there it can work out the contribution it can make in different arenas:

- *Neighbourhoods* which are being destroyed as a result of the interacting processes of decline: high unemployment, widespread poverty, sub-standard housing, a deteriorating environment, fear, mistrust, high mobility, etc.
- *Networks* of people who share a similar identity, problem or interest – for example, those who have the same faith, people who have the same

housing tenure, parents of children at risk of drug misuse, victims of crime, etc. This way of understanding 'community', particularly as it relates to race, sexuality and gender, challenges much of the practice wisdom in community development.

* *Agencies* such as local authorities which have the capacity to respond strategically to economic and social problems in their areas. Community development can play a key role within such a framework. In the British context the experience of Strathclyde Regional Council from 1976 stands as an important source of information in this context – when we examine the French context we shall see that there is comparable material on strategic community development.

* *Policies* of government and the European Union which impinge directly upon the lives of people living in deprived communities and which can be influenced by community development ideas and experiences.)

If the starting point for community development is for it to position itself across these arenas in relation to an analysis of poverty, inequality and powerlessness, then the need for it to respond to the situation of children surely becomes unanswerable:

* (*Poverty.* The numbers of children and young people in the poorest families have increased rapidly. In 1979, 1.4 million dependent children were living in households with incomes below half the national average; in 1990/91 the figure was 3.9 million, an increase from one-tenth to one-third of the age group. The extent of child poverty has been confirmed more recently by the major report on poverty and wealth in the UK published by the Joseph Rowntree Foundation (Barclay 1995).

* *Environment.* There is increasing evidence of the effects on children's health of traffic and other pollutants, as well as of the risks of accidents caused by the expansion of car ownership.

* *Safety.* Children no longer feel as safe in public places as they used to – hence the increase in journeys by car to school and elsewhere. Fear of attack, danger from traffic, concerns about drugs and crime are the key factors.)

(The effects of poverty, environment and fear are to deny children the rights they should have to exist and play in neighbourhoods. This statement provides the opposite picture to media portrayals of some neighbourhoods as being under the control of children and young people – in this scenario it is the adults who are the victims: 10-year-olds harassing adult residents and riot situations developing.)

Where does the truth lie in this conflicting portrayal of children's lives in neighbourhoods? We have to look for the answer, it seems to me, in the value society puts, or does not put, on children and their need to develop and express themselves. When children and young people riot (Campbell 1993) or when pranks go wrong and cause injury or death, it is surely because children feel that they have been let down by adults.

We are in danger of cutting off ways in which adults can communicate and undertake joint activities with children outside home and institutional settings. In many areas resources for youth work, playschemes and adventure playgrounds have been reduced to an alarming extent. There appears to be a retreat by policy makers from supporting local people at the local neighbourhood level in terms of building relationships between people, especially those between children and adults. Ironically the experience of community workers is that the motivation of adults to become involved in community activities which benefit children directly is normally very strong. Hasler shows how important it is for community workers to take up children's issues and to avoid using them as a means of simply getting at the adults: 'The challenge is to see children and young people as part of the community in their own right' (Hasler 1995: 181).

This challenge needs to be taken up by a number of professions, particularly social work, education and youth work, and in terms of how practitioners and managers seek to work with children. Community development has the experience, knowledge and skills to contribute to such a developmental process so that, at the same time as it puts forward the case for more work to be done with children, it can also show what that work might look like and specify the knowledge and skills needed for it to be effective.

WORKING WITH CHILDREN

Community development 'reconstructed' so as to work more seriously, strategically and skilfully with children would need to make at least two paradigmatic shifts:

• a move away from a narrow social work interpretation of the phrase 'working with children';
• a move towards integration with economic and regeneration programmes.

Advocates of these shifts (to which we return in the chapter's final section) can draw upon a significant cluster of practice experiences, research and policy evidence to support their case. Some practice experiences are included and referenced in *Children and Communities* (Henderson 1995). Another key resource is the writings of Holman (1981, 1996) who has made a unique contribution to this area because he has combined the roles of practitioner, writer and theoretician. Both of these are the tip of the iceberg in terms of practice experiences across the UK over a period of more than twenty years: a few are recorded in case-study form, most are held in the memories of the community workers and local people involved.

In terms of research there is now important material contained in reports on family centres, especially those which have adopted an open-access, neighbourhood-based approach. Teresa Smith's study of six family projects run by The Children's Society found that 'Given the levels of disadvantage evident in many areas, "open access" and support for community resources is likely in the long run to benefit more families as part of a preventive neighbourhood-based strategy not restricted to referred families' (Smith 1993: 10). Research by Gibbons leads her to state that family projects had 'strengthened local community resources, by providing new activities and advice points, by drawing in new volunteers, and by opening up new opportunities for local people' (Gibbons 1990: 158). And Owen Gill has shown how research into child protection is pointing to the need for a neighbourhood-based approach:

> There should be more emphasis on working to support and strengthen those neighbourhoods which produce high rates of child protection cases. Such work would be based on the approaches of bringing people together, developing a sense of neighbourhood identity, articulating the demands for resources, and playing a part in creating the complex criss-crossing of relationships which is the sign of a mature and supportive community.
>
> (Gill 1995: 30)

The international research led by Quortrup (1991) into childhood, as well as research findings from children's projects in developing countries (see Boyden 1991), are also key sources.

The policy aspects of children and neighbourhoods are to be found most obviously in the policy statements and strategy documents of the four main child care voluntary organisations – The Children's Society, Barnardo's, NCH Action for Children and Save the Children. All of these, in varying degrees, have committed themselves to a neighbourhood-based approach to working with children and families. A small number of local authorities have demonstrated an interest in moving in that direction.

Experiences in France

In addition to making use of practice, research and policy developments to develop a clearer idea of the community development agenda for working with children, it is appropriate to examine approaches in France. This comparative exercise is done at this point in order to help sharpen the points for a UK debate, albeit that the French situation is also of interest in its own right.

At the macro, national level it is the French experience of decentralisation and government commitment to a major programme of urban social development that is of interest to community development commentators in the UK. Crescy Cannan shows how the Développement Social des Quartiers (DSQ), launched by the mayor of Grenoble in 1982, has led to the emergence of 'new complex relations of power. Local actors have been mobilised to work together' (Cannan 1995: 238–47).

Three aspects of the DSQ are especially relevant to community development. First, it has encouraged flexibility and innovation at the local level. For example, at a London seminar held in 1992 to learn about French urban and social policy, participants heard how a judge at Strasbourg's juvenile courts initiated new, neighbourhood-based methods in a district of the city:

> The holding of a civil hearing in the area will lesson the divide which exists between those sections of the population which are experiencing most problems and a system of justice which they resent and regard as being hostile and alien to them.
>
> (Beau 1989: 1)

This particular project lasted for eight years and was run in conjunction with the local commission of the DSQ.

The second important feature of the DSQ as far as community development is concerned has been its promotion of the policy of *insertion* (integration). This is because, although the major thrust of *insertion* is to increase the possibilities for unemployed people to enter the labour market, it also recognises the importance of *social* integration:

> It thus implies policies, resulting in extensive socio-cultural services from centres for youth, families and children, and so forth, working to promote harmonious relationships between groups, generations, races, and contributing to civic consciousness and active citizenship.
>
> (Cannan 1995: 238–47)

Finally, the DSQ is able to encourage and fund programmes which are essentially preventive. There have been strong pressures to try and break

down barriers between professions and most of the prevention programmes have been concerned with anti-delinquency measures, notably
extensive holiday schemes for children and young people.

A similar interest in encouraging different groups of professionals to
work together more effectively is discernible in the social work and
community work sectors. Social workers, *animateurs socio-culturels*
(centre-based community workers) and *éducateurs specialisés* (near-
equivalent to detached youth workers), all of whom receive their
own separate professional training, appear to be more prepared than
previously to learn from each other and to work together. The membership organisation for those people who have a co-ordinating role in
districts (*responsables de circonscription*) remains dominated by social
workers but includes *animateurs* and *éducateurs*. Some years ago it
changed its name to Movement for Local Social Development (described
in Marie-Renée Bourget-Daitch and Chris Warren's chapter in this
volume).

The other feature of French social work with and on behalf of children
which relates to community development is the use of state agency
contracts for work with children and families. The government circular
of 26 June 1984 on '*le contrat famille*' puts an emphasis on prevention,
co-ordination, inter-professionalism and innovation and a number of
commentators believe that it contains considerable scope for imaginative
social planning on the part of elected members, practitioners, community
groups and users.

Since 1988 the '*contrats enfance*' have encouraged local authorities
to promote a holistic approach to the care of young children (up to 6 years
old). Arguably this policy has been introduced as much in response to
the needs of working parents as to the needs of children. However, there
can be no doubt of the considerable political and professional commitment behind it. It has resulted in the growth of a variety of nurseries, play
centres, after-school clubs and day centres. By 1992 more than 1,000
contracts were in existence.

The other important development in France in the context of children
and communities has been the growth of children's councils. Linked to
local authorities, there are now more than 700 of these forums in the
country. They provide an opportunity for local authority representatives
to listen to the ideas and suggestions of children. While clearly of limited
value in terms of relating to children in neighbourhoods, the councils
illustrate an official recognition of the need for children to have ways of
expressing opinions to a degree that is not matched in Britain.

What points emerge for our discussion of community development and children from this brief look at UK practice, research and policy experiences and at social development and social work in France? And in what ways could they inform community development work with and on behalf of children?

Policy

The importance of there being a policy framework within which children-focused community development can take place is very evident. Compared with the resources and sense of direction arising from the French DSQ, initiatives in the UK have the feel of being a hotchpotch of projects which have been dependent upon the flair and energy of individuals and the capacity to tap research and project funds.

It is enterprise, training for employment and investment that are the watchwords of national and regional policies in the UK, not children. There is little sign of government departments developing joint policies on behalf of children. The Department of Health, Department of the Environment, Department for Education and Employment and the Home Office all have key responsibilities for children. A serious policy commitment to working on their behalf would surely need to ensure that departments were working together – and could be seen to be doing so.

Accessibility

Community development work with and on behalf of children needs to operate on a small scale if it is to be meaningful. Using a geographical unit any larger than a neighbourhood is likely to result in a distancing of the very people – children and adults – with whom community development seeks to engage. It would be like expecting all primary school children to attend one large institution, using the same catchment area as for a secondary school.

If we are serious about the involvement of children and young people in community activities and action, and commitment to their participation in decision making, then safe, accessible lines of communication are essential. This is a recurrent theme in Bob Holman's case study of a neighbourhood project on the Easterhouse estate, Glasgow: the advantages of both voluntary and statutory staff being near to local people, aware of the problems they face and being available to listen (Holman 1996).

De-mystification

In an interesting reversal of the supposedly contrasting differences of approach by the British and French (the former favouring pragmatism and empiricism, the latter theorising and abstraction), British material on community development tends to emphasise processes of empowerment whereas the French face in the direction of services and activities. Both approaches are, of course, needed. The importance, however, of having clear, jargon-free language, given that children are the focal point, must be paramount.

There is an opportunity to claim the ground for a new, de-mystified dialogue: how adults and children talk about the neighbourhoods where they live, the potential contribution of community development work with and on behalf of children. A determination to operate in this way would be a refreshing contrast to much of the North American dominated language surrounding regeneration, capacity building and partnerships.

It is as much about how things are done as what is done, and this is an approach which is embedded deeply in community development values: the importance of working within the experiences and culture of local people; making sure that people are not further disempowered as a result of the language and timescales demanded so often by external agencies; and making sure that the voices of children themselves are heard: they will bring a directness, concreteness and authenticity to the discussions which will help ground these in the realities of community life.

Contracts

The idea of a contract between several parties has a sharper connotation than 'partnership' or even 'agreement'. The growth of children's services and facilities in France has come from the state, and the use of contracts has bound together the state, local authorities and – to a lesser degree – communities.

Policy makers in Britain who are responsible for encouraging partnerships between the various sectors and who are keen to ensure that communities are not marginalised could see contracts as a useful additional tool. In a sense the state, in the French context, is setting out comparative definitions of need and using a mixture of carrot and stick to encourage local authorities to make improvements in the interests of children (this is also discussed by Cresy Cannan in Chapter 4). As a result, national standards can be used alongside local requirements.

The notion of contracts, therefore, between localities and the state could be beneficial to an active community development approach to working with and on behalf of children. The experience of partnerships in Britain underlines the need for practitioners to support community groups in negotiations and decision making about resources.

A NEW BEGINNING?

The statement was made earlier that children are affected by a number of forces in neighbourhoods. These include the physical environment, breakdown of communication between children and adults, fear and conflicts within communities, and commercial and media pressures. It is this multiplicity of factors that must be recognised by agencies. Only then will a truly 'rounded' and strategic approach emerge. Backward-looking perspectives are not needed. The debate must shift away from the framework and concerns of one profession or discipline and towards an analysis that takes the situation of children and communities as the starting point.

Community development has to engage more with the issue of children's needs in deprived neighbourhoods. Ideally one would like to see a similar level of energy and commitment being injected as has happened with research and campaigning on children's rights in recent years. Those Articles of the UN Convention on the Rights of the Child which relate to children's participation could be picked up and used in imaginative ways by advocates of community development: right to express opinions (Article 12), right to freedom of expression (Article 13), right to associate freely (Article 15) and right to play (Article 31).

Yet other building blocks will need to be put in place if effective community development work with children is to happen. Each of the three following themes requires to be clarified and strengthened if, together, they are to offer a sufficiently robust basis on which to sustain children-focused community development.

Integrating the social and economic

Finding ways whereby the 'social' aspects of communities are genuinely taken seriously within regeneration programmes will not be easy. The hold of powerful organisations whose main priority is economic development of one form or another is considerable. In a number of local authorities, however, there is an awareness of the need to make and support connections between the economic and social, as well as to ensure that authentic consultation processes are put in place.

Examples of what is meant by the social aspects of regeneration are:

- community-based crime and drug prevention programmes;
- resources for children's play areas, with active involvement of children and adults in their design, location and management;
- neighbourhood centres which, depending on local need, can provide a mix of advice, information, meeting point, safety, etc.;
- plans and resources for elderly people, people with learning disabilities and other vulnerable groups who live in the community but who are often isolated and stigmatised.

At one level, the introduction of these kinds of social issues into regeneration programmes will add to the complexity of working in communities because conflicting priorities and points of view will become more evident: intermediate technology training for young people or leisure activities for elderly people? Traffic-free zones for child safety or easy access for plant vehicles etc.?

Yet at another level such an approach offers a more sensitive and 'rounded' approach to communities. Not only does it take the long-term view, it also recognises the breadth and variety of human need and how this has to constitute the essence of 'community'.

Realistically it may be that regeneration programmes cannot be 'turned' far enough in the direction outlined above. Attempts must be made to do so, but the programmes may already be too strongly established and the vested interests too immovable. A parallel strategy is to work within the framework of social exclusion programmes. Here the opportunities available to inject social issues are more evident.

Increasing numbers of local authorities in Britain now have active anti-poverty strategies. Researchers studying these developments point to the importance of strategies including a strong community development element: 'In terms of anti-poverty strategic development, we have little doubt . . . that community involvement in the local decision-making process could be greatly enhanced' (Alcock *et al.* 1995: 73–4).

Social exclusion is being recognised as a key concept by increasing numbers of policy makers and politicians within Europe (despite the European Union's Council of Ministers' refusal in June 1995 to proceed with a successor to the European Anti-Poverty Programme, Poverty 3). The European Anti-Poverty Network has established itself as a respected lobby within the European Union, and anti-poverty organisations in several countries are making important connections between anti-poverty work and community development – the Irish organisation, Combat Poverty Agency, and Scotland's Poverty Alliance being good examples.

Social exclusion emphasises the multi-dimensional nature of the problem. On the one hand, community development offers a tangible way whereby people, acting together, can achieve more control over basic aspects of their lives – through food co-operatives and credit unions, for example. On the other hand, community development principles of empowerment and learning can underpin such activities.

The potential of campaigning organisations to make links with community development principles and organisations is considerable:

> Community development, with its fundamental emphasis on the participation and empowerment of the poor, reminds us that there is a need constantly to recreate other ways of living and making decisions about the distribution of material, cultural and social resources.
>
> (Craig 1994: 8, paper 2)

Placing children at the centre of social inclusion strategies that contain a significant community development element should be paramount. Such an approach opens up creative opportunities to combine income-related work for children and their families with initiatives aimed at facilitating the positive involvement of children in neighbourhoods. The urgency to develop such a twin-track approach is obvious to anyone who has witnessed either the effects of child poverty or the negative consequences of failing to address children's needs in neighbourhoods – or both.

Building alliances

For community development involving children to take root in both policy and practice terms it is essential that organisations work together more effectively:

Voluntary child care organisations

The Children's Society, Save the Children, Barnardo's, and NCH Action for Children already work on the issue of children and community. There is surely similar scope within the National Society for the Prevention of Cruelty to Children and other child care organisations. Equally important is for stronger links to be made between these organisations and children's play organisations. And those churches committed to using community development methods, perhaps as a result of Church Urban Fund projects, are likely to be interested in making connections with organisations on the issue of children. The Church and Neighbourhood

Action projects of Barnardo's are an example of how 'children' and 'community' can be brought together in this way.

A further dimension to a discussion of alliance building among organisations is to test the extent to which organisations that focus on the family are interested in engaging with the issue of children's 'community'. The impression is that it has not been on their agendas in a substantive way to date.

Children's rights

The energy of organisations such as the Children's Rights Development Unit can be drawn upon by advocates of community development and children. The UN Convention on the Rights of the Child means that there is an important international dimension to such work.

Local authorities

Anti-poverty strategies of local authorities are supported by two national organisations, the Local Government Anti-Poverty Unit and the National Local Government Forum Against Poverty, and these offer tangible opportunities to raise the issue of children in the context of community development. So too do the Local Agenda 21 initiatives of local authorities in the sphere of children and the environment.

The other area requiring development is local authorities' interpretation of the Children Act 1989. The Act's intention was that prevention of child abuse should run in parallel with protection. So far, however, both social services departments and – more surprisingly – social work departments in Scotland – have been slow to develop the former. The Department of Health-commissioned research (1995) may provide a chink of light for change to occur here: a wider perspective on child protection and the development of services that would enhance children's general quality of life are identified as two preconditions of effective practice.

Community groups and children

For the issue of community development and children really to achieve political purchase within national and local social policy debates it is essential that community groups and children be included in alliance building. This is easier said than done. Money and time are needed to achieve it and the likelihood is that the professional organisations will tend to be dominant in terms of the language used, the priorities set and the pace at which action is taken.

Perhaps the most reliable way of including community groups and children is to argue for it to be part of best professional practice. A process that achieves in the sphere of children and communities what user involvement has gained in the community care field is needed: an assumption that communities and children will participate rather than that they would if better conditions prevailed.

Community development experience tells us that we should be optimistic rather than pessimistic here: adults are prepared to struggle for a better future for their children and interpreting this only in individual or family terms is generally recognised as being insufficient. Children need good quality play areas and safe streets, community centres should not be monopolised by adults, etc. and it is possible to locate the energy and commitment among adults to help achieve these things. On this basis there is every likelihood that they will see that it is important to work with others at regional and national levels as well as with children at neighbourhood level.

Efforts – such as those described by Jenny Clifton and David Hodgson in Chapter 2 – made by children and community groups to develop regional and national networks on the issue of children and neighbour-hoods and to forge links with professional organisations must be supported. Such a push from the grassroots would undoubtedly be a key factor in taking the wider debate forward.

Knowledge and skills

During a seminar on children and communities one participant expressed scepticism about the role of community development because he felt it was such an adult concept; it could never really understand children.

It is true that community development is not equipped to provide psychological insight into children's thinking and behaviour. This is the province of other disciplines and professions. Community development's contribution lies in the knowledge and skills it can bring to bear on the processes of groups which are acting in the public domain. Accordingly it has had to develop its own body of knowledge and skills which cross-cuts between group work and research theory, political science and social policy.

At the core of community work practice/theory are the ideas of enabling and facilitation, and the community worker's role has been identified very much on this basis. He or she works in communities and supports community groups with the aim of bringing about change. Process models which specify the worker's role and identify the required skill and knowledge areas have been developed (Henderson and Thomas 1987; Twelvetrees 1991).

The theme of children and community development must inevitably be critical of this body of practice/theory because (a) there is a need to respond to the rapidly changing contexts of policies and communities in the mid-1990s, (b) there is a need to maximise the use of new techniques and methods which have been found to be effective by community workers and others, and (c) we need to work effectively with and on behalf of children in their neighbourhoods. Accordingly we are looking to identify skills and knowledge which, while drawing upon previous experiences of practice and training, are alert to the new context I have argued for in this chapter. There is space only to put forward three ideas in response to this challenge:

Social policy

Advocates and practitioners of community development and children need to acquire a body of knowledge about children and society which is inter-disciplinary and which draws upon research evidence. Only in this way will it be possible to make inroads into professional de-marcations and traditions. At present, this knowledge base is generally weak among both practitioners and managers; they appear not to make use of research and policy material relating to children and communities which has been generated in Britain and elsewhere in recent years.

One illustration to make the point: in 1993 the Eisenhower Foundation identified Head Start pre-schools as an example of the kind of programme that should be supported by the US government, citing evaluations that Head Start is 'perhaps the most cost-effective across-the-board inner city prevention strategy ever developed'. How many practitioners and managers in Britain are aware of this and ready to use it in policy and strategy discussions, to argue for neighbourhood-based programmes?

Community practice

There is evidence to suggest that, while the number of generalist community workers in Britain may have declined over the last twelve years, the number of practitioners – fieldwork staff across a range of agencies whose jobs contain a significant 'community' element – has increased. Small-scale studies undertaken by Bradford & Ilkley Community College included a survey of paid practitioners in Bradford. A total of 246 practitioners were identified (Glen 1993). Between them they covered fourteen policy areas and the types of community practice ranged from self-help and cultural activities to campaigning and advocacy, developing services and resources, training and research/ information. The studies also included a review of the community policies of public agencies in West Yorkshire, and a survey of nationally advertised posts in community practice. Both of these indicate more extensive recruitment of community practitioners by statutory agencies across a range of policy fields.

If there is a trend towards community practice in ways indicated above, then it is essential that practice/theory is developed which takes account of the fact that work with communities constitutes only part of many practitioners' jobs: health workers, community economic development staff, crime prevention officers, social workers, youth workers, etc. The implications in terms of re-assessing the knowledge and skills required by such people to engage with the issue of children in communities are likely to be considerable.

Local education . . . preventive strategies

Practitioners who are committed to extending community development work with and on behalf of children would be well advised to seek support from community practitioners focusing on other issues. The idea of 'local education' as discussed by Mark Smith is helpful here. He suggests that use of the term can help to identify the interactions between individuals and institutions in specific localities. It brings out the significance of local knowledge:

> This means that local educators do not make use of a formal curriculum for much of their work. They work in settings not usually associated with education. Much of their conversation, as a result, is not immediately distinguishable from what might be said between friends or neighbours.
>
> (Smith 1994: 161)

Thinking of community practitioners as local educators opens up the possibility of identifying core knowledge and skill areas amongst social workers, youth workers, educators and other practitioners who work in communities. As well as placing community development and children within a cluster of generic knowledge and skill areas, the concept of 'local education' also gives support to the theme of prevention: the common components of crime prevention, delinquency prevention, drug abuse prevention, etc. These practice areas will be strengthened immeasurably if they can be shown to share common skills and knowledge about working in and with communities.

I am suggesting, therefore, that neighbourhood work knowledge and skills need to be re-assessed from a theoretical perspective, and that making connections with a number of different types of practice may be the key to establishing such a perspective. Community development work with children would undoubtedly benefit.

CONCLUDING COMMENTS

A new beginning is needed, and in this chapter a number of building blocks have been identified to show how a new start can be made. Underlying them is the vision of a welfare state that eschews an overly economistic and individualistic view of citizenship. Rather, it is a vision that rediscovers the profound significance of all people being treated as people and of the value of co-operative and collective forms of human activity.

In such a society children would be of more central importance than they are today – 'A touchstone of the health and strength of a society' (Commission on Social Justice 1994: 310). The concept of welfare would be broader, with professionals motivated and equipped to work more substantively both with each other and with communities. Within such a scenario it would be important for community development to continue to play a role that is both innovatory and challenging.

REFERENCES

Alcock, P., Craig, G., Dalgleish, K. and Pearson, S. (1995) *Combating Local Poverty*, Luton: Local Government Management Board.

Barclay, P. (1995) *Joseph Rowntree Foundation Inquiry into Income and Wealth*, York: Joseph Rowntree Foundation.

Beau, C. (1989) 'Eight years of judicial practice at Neuhof', Strasbourg: mimeo.

Boyden, J. (1991) *Children of the Cities*, London: Zed Books.

Campbell, B. (1993) *Goliath – Britain's Dangerous Places*, London: Methuen.

Cannan, C. (1995) 'Urban social development in France', *Community Development Journal*, 30, 3: 238–47.

Commission on Social Justice (1994) *Social Justice – Strategies for National Renewal*, London: Vintage.

Craig, G. (1994) 'Social exclusion and community development', in *Policy for Practice*, Glasgow: Scottish Community Development Centre.

Department of Health (1995) *Child Protection: Messages From Research*, London: HMSO.

Gibbons, J. (1990) *Family Support and Prevention: Studies in Local Areas*, London: NISW/HMSO.

Gill, O. (1995) 'Neighbourhood watch', *Community Care*, 8–14 June 1995.

Glen, A. (1993) 'Methods and themes in community practice', in H. Butcher, A. Glen, P. Henderson and J. Smith (eds), *Community and Public Policy*, London: Pluto Press.

Hasler, J. (1995) 'Belonging and becoming: the child growing up in community', in P. Henderson (ed.), *Children and Communities*, London: Pluto Press in association with CDF/The Children's Society.

Henderson, P. (ed.) (1995) *Children and Communities*, London: Pluto Press in association with CDF/The Children's Society.

Henderson, P. and Thomas, D. N. (1987) *Skills in Neighbourhood Work*, London: Allen & Unwin.

Holman, B. (1981) *Kids at the Door*, Oxford: Basil Blackwell.

Holman, B. (1996) 'Fare dealing', unpublished paper, Glasgow.

Quortrup, (1991) *Children as a Social Phenomenon: An Introduction to a Series of National Reports*, Vienna: European Centre for Social Welfare Policy and Research.

Smith, M. (1994) *Local Education*, Buckingham: Open University Press.

Smith, T. (1993) 'Family centres and bringing up young children', Oxford: Department of Applied Social Studies and Social Research (mimeo).

Thomas, D. (1995) *Community Development at Work*, London: CDF/Joseph Rowntree Foundation.

Twelvetrees, A. (1991) *Community Work*, Basingstoke: Macmillan.

Chapter 2

Rethinking practice through a children's rights perspective

Jenny Clifton and David Hodgson

Children are overlooked when it comes to decision making. Many people will argue that children are not mature or experienced enough to have anything to offer, but when these decisions affect us why shouldn't we be entitled to an opinion?

(ROC 1995)[1]

In recent years the issue of children's rights has gained a prominence not only in the arena of child care and social work but also in terms of popular culture. While opinions vary about the significance of legislative changes heralded by the Children Act 1989 in terms of progress towards recognition of children's rights, few commentators would disagree that it holds out the prospect of a more central position for children with regard to decisions made by courts and local authorities, if not within the family more generally. This chapter will consider the implications of this apparent trend towards greater acknowledgement of rights for children for those working in the local state. Activities based on a children's rights perspective, in which both younger and older people play a significant part, have created real opportunities not only to review practice with children but more broadly to reappraise the relationship between children, families and communities. It is suggested that a children's rights perspective can contribute to a reassessment of strategies for family support and child protection, can highlight the potential for involving children and young people in decisions affecting their lives and is an essential aspect of a 'social action' approach to welfare practice.

This chapter explores the concept of children's rights and strategies at the levels of both policy and practice which are intended to empower young people. Many of the ideas discussed here were developed as a result of working with the group of young people involved in a Young People's Festival of Rights and since it is central to this chapter that children's perspectives are heard and taken seriously, their words illustrate many of the themes. The chapter concludes with reflection on the implications of these strategies for welfare professionals. The terms 'children' and 'young people' have been used somewhat interchangeably, to refer to those under the age of majority.

CHILDREN'S RIGHTS: SOME PERSPECTIVES

Before exploring the practical implications of a concern for children's rights, it is important to reflect on the concept itself.

What do children mean by rights?

Children of primary school age demonstrate an awareness of rights in moral terms and they increasingly develop an understanding of the universality of rights. In one research project Norwegian children showed particular concerns for positive rights, their comments reflecting their political and cultural context:

> (12 year old boy) 'Everyone has the right to free health and health service.'
> (13 year old girl) 'Peace, care, food, clothes and education.'
> (Melton and Limber 1992: 178)

When consulted about their perception of rights, young people involved in the ROC Festival raised many concerns, including homelessness, criminal justice legislation and the environment. They emphasised their wish to play a part in influencing decision making on such issues alongside adults.

Contributions from rights theorists

There is a tendency to talk of children's rights as if they were completely separate from human rights more generally. In fact, the first recorded global declaration of human rights concerned not adults but children. The Declaration of the Rights of the Child was unanimously adopted by the League of Nations in 1924. The concept of rights symbolises fundamental beliefs about treating people as human beings. In Freeman's words, rights entitle individuals 'to respect and dignity: no amount of benevolence or compassion can be an adequate substitute' (Freeman 1992: 29). Rights, according to Freeman, are based on two fundamental principles. First, the principle of equality and equal concern for each person – rights outlaw prejudice and discrimination, declaring all individuals to be equal before the law; second, rights are derived from the principle of autonomy – not a declaration of absolute freedom to do exactly as we would wish but a recognition of individual integrity and self-respect together with respect for others. Rights concern entitlement, claims and respect and the protection of interests, needs and capacities essential for 'human flourishing' (Freeden 1991: 9).

Approaches based on rights have been criticised from a variety of standpoints, particularly when applied to children. Concern has been expressed about an overemphasis on legal remedies and a preoccupation with individualism, even self-centredness in the language of rights. The discussion in this chapter utilises a rights perspective which does not rely on legalism and is founded on a much broader humanism. Its objectives are entirely consistent with concerns about communities as well as individuals and, indeed, entail a recognition of interdependency and mutuality between adults and young people and between young people themselves (Archard 1993; Eekelaar 1992).

The concept of rights has contributed towards a re-evaluation of childhood in at least three ways. First, it represents a shift away from a definition of childhood solely in terms of 'needs', thereby moving away from a preoccupation with problem-centred dependency and towards a recognition of universal claims which children themselves help to articulate (see Boushel and Lebacq 1992). Second, the existence of the United Nations Convention on the Rights of the Child 1989 (UNCRC) has helped to clarify the moral foundation for children's rights, representing as it does a fundamental challenge to divisions between civil and political rights, and economic and social rights (McGoldrick 1991). The Convention requires a re-evaluation of all legislation, policy and practice affecting children and implies the conversion of the moral claims of childhood into specific legal rights (Alston *et al.* 1992, 1994; Freeman and Veerman 1992).

Third, rights theorists have made an effective case for the recognition of rights for children on the basis that they, like adults, have specific 'interests' – in particular concerning care and nurture – and are entitled to respect as persons (Eekelaar 1986). Beyond this, however, children have their own 'project interests' – their own agenda of concerns often not shared by adults and easily overlooked by them (Wolfson 1992). This notion of 'interests' is a particularly helpful way of thinking about children's place in the community. The planning of the ROC Festival represented a concerted attempt to define not just the issues for debate, but the actual shape of the event by finding out what young people wanted to say and how they wanted to say it. As a consequence of young people taking the lead role in organising the event, the topics were broad and were approached not just through discussion but through representation in music, craft and drama.

Liberation versus protection: polarised perceptions of children and rights

Debates about children's rights have often been presented in terms of apparently irreconcilable extremes by contrasting notions of protection and liberation. A protectionist approach to children's rights views childhood itself as the basis for asserting special interests and protective measures for a particularly vulnerable group of human beings. The liberationist view was founded on the notion of childhood as merely a social construct that denied civil and political rights using the arbitrary criterion of age. In this view, children should be allowed access to the same rights as adults (see Fox Harding 1991).

Discussion of these contrasting perceptions may assist an exploration of social policy in respect of children: it can be said, for example, that much current child care law and policy is founded on a form of protectionism which tends to undermine rather than support children's rights or, at least, to reduce rights to a 'default' measure 'exercisable only when parents . . . fail in their responsibilities' (Smith 1991: 478). Such discussion can also usefully address the negative impact of adult views of children's competence. For Archard, a valuable insight of the child liberationists is their observation that while children are presumed incompetent, they are unlikely to be given opportunities either to develop or to demonstrate competence (Archard 1993: 68). Research on children's grasp of controversial issues suggests that adults often underestimate children's awareness and knowledge (Short 1988).

However, one of the problems of polarisation in discussion of children's rights is that it can reinforce popular myths, for example the view that to give children rights is to agree to whatever they want and that this is what children are seeking. Such assumptions only serve to obscure the views and wishes of children. A more helpful view is offered by Freeman:

Children who are not protected, whose welfare is not advanced, will not be able to exercise self-determination; on the other hand, a failure to recognise the personality of children is likely to result in an undermining of their protection with children reduced to objects of intervention.

(Freeman 1993a: 42)

A more holistic approach to children's rights, avoiding the pitfalls of either extreme view, can contribute to a re-evaluation of the adult role in facilitating the development of young people's autonomy. Before this theme is developed further, it is important to consider the relevance of the concept of rights to the everyday experience of children.

Rights and power

There is a close relationship between concepts of rights and of power. Genuine shifts in power relationships are necessary for access to rights to become a reality for children and this is why discussions of rights must include the practical empowerment of children (Frost and Stein 1989). Children have little formal power and are largely dependent on adults to represent and protect their interests. Within the family, while policy statements often seem to assume that the interests of parents and children naturally coincide, some parents clearly do not have the best interests of their children at heart. The relevance of power relations to the study of child abuse and to the experience of women and children in the family is receiving increasing recognition, though more attention needs to be given to the different experiences of boys and girls (Parton 1990; McNay 1992; Segal 1995). There will be conflicts of interests between family members and some hold more power than others. The exercise of such power is structured by age and by gender and the two are linked, as the evidence on male violence to women and children shows (Mullender and Morley 1994). Ennew (1986) comments that women too may oppress children and limit their rights in the name of 'knowing best'. In a feminist critique of the UN Convention, Olsen (1992) has highlighted the complex interaction between women's rights and children's rights and in so doing has clearly defined the kind of conflicts that may arise.

Except in Scotland[2] there is no general legal provision in the UK for children to be involved in decisions within the family. Opportunities under the Children Act 1989 for children to apply to the courts, while of symbolic significance, are highly circumscribed and inappropriate for most family situations (CRDU 1994: 23). What of children's daily experience of family decision making? When a group of children aged 10 to 12 talked about relationships with their parents, they emphasised the importance of respect, which included being taken seriously and being treated fairly (Hodgson 1994). When parents explained the restrictions on their children's freedom or gradually and explicitly allowed them more responsibility the children felt respected. There was a strong sense of what was 'fair' and 'unfair' behaviour between adults and children, particularly when it came to sibling treatment. Children wanted a say in deciding punishments, to be given some privacy, and above all wanted to be believed. Their desire and need for support from their parents was evident. They did not demand to take over responsibility for themselves but wanted discussion and negotiation about the rules.

The children provided examples of disrespectful treatment from parents:

'They switch on and off about you';
'They talk to their friends about you ... show you up ... slag you off';
'You have to say please but they never do';
'They don't realise we have feelings. Like when I cried when my dog died and Dad asked why I was being a baby.'

(Hodgson 1994)

Other dimensions of power require a brief mention. As yet, discussions of children's rights have tended to be as ungendered as those concerned with 'need' or 'protection', but there is literature on girls' experience of care and of the criminal justice system which highlights the impact of sexism in policy and practice (Carlen and Wardhaugh 1991). The complex interaction between forms of power can result in multiple oppressions: for black children the consequences of racism, both personal and institutional, impact on their access to rights (Modi *et al.* 1995). Finally, professionals who work with children need to address their own use of power and the way in which 'professional expertise' may undermine children's views by reference to their welfare or best interests.

Rethinking paternalism

Some commentators have addressed the concern that to permit children to exercise complete freedom of decision making might result in their most fundamental interests being damaged, through lack of knowledge or the maturity to make decisions that would further their long-term interests. For Eekelaar (1994), this potential to jeopardise one's future justifies a form of paternalism which is rooted in developmental notions of autonomy. This would require that adults provide an environment in which children can fully develop their potential for contributing to decision making throughout childhood. He uses the concept of 'dynamic self-determinism' to encompass the evolving nature of the child's contribution to the outcome of decisions.

Freeman's (1983) model of 'liberal paternalism' requires the justification of adult interference with the child's self-determination, encompassing a notion of 'future-oriented consent' (Dworkin 1971: 119). Legitimate actions would be those enabling the child to grow into full adulthood and those that the future adult might understand. Both Eekelaar and Freeman suggest models of 'substituted judgement' to permit maximum recognition of the child's wishes, feelings and experience in contributing to decisions about their lives. These would engage adult decision makers in a process of projection, based on a thorough knowledge of that child, concerning what the child might want were he or she able to direct his or her affairs, rather than simply deciding what is best from the adults' own perspective on what children need.

Such models are concerned with creating space for the exercise of autonomous decision making by children within the context of protecting and promoting their longer-term interests. Though helpful, they appear to derive from an adult-oriented view of decision making primarily concerned with individual welfare. In contrast, the concept of children's 'project interests' is useful to a consideration of how adults may empower children to participate in matters affecting their lives and which reflect their own agenda of concerns. In the early meetings to plan the ROC Festival adults were surprised at the breadth of issues children wanted to raise and their awareness of how their own immediate concerns linked to major issues, for example in respect of the law and the environment. The issue for the adults became one of how best to provide the context for developing this potential contribution.

This debate about paternalism has implications for the role of the state in the care of children. It has been suggested that the state is at present relating to children in a traditionally paternalistic way, largely seeking to re-create the parent–child relationship though at a greater psychological distance from the child (Bell 1993). A children's rights perspective points to the need to reappraise the respective positions of children, parents and the state and, in particular, to forge a new relationship between children and the state which regards them as citizens worthy of respect rather than potentially victims or villains. This does not necessarily imply an antagonistic relationship with parents. However, it does involve recognition of children's claims on both parents and the state.

PROTECTION AND PARTICIPATION: ISSUES AND STRATEGIES

> No social organisation can hope to be built on the rights of its members unless there are mechanisms whereby those members may express themselves and wherein those expressions are taken seriously. *Hearing what children say* must therefore lie at the root of any elaboration of children's rights.
>
> (Eekelaar 1992: 228; Eekelaar's italics)

The preceding discussion of perspectives on children's rights has already pointed to links between protection, welfare, autonomy and participation. The following section will consider how a rights perspective can help to reframe approaches to protection and how children can contribute to the definition of their own welfare through various forms of participation.

The most comprehensive statement of the current position on children's rights in the UK is the 'Agenda for Children', an appraisal of law, policy and practice against the standards of the UN Convention on the Rights of the Child (CRDU 1994). The authors highlight the significance of Article 12, which gives children the right to participate in all decisions affecting them. This is the starting point for the following attempt to explore new notions of child care. A variety of research and action projects have contributed to an understanding of how children's voices can be heard, and some of these will be drawn upon in the following discussion[3]. More research is needed which explores children's evaluations of their interactions with adults.

The rights perspective offers three ways of reframing the protection of children, each suggesting ways in which children's views can become more influential. First there is a broader, holistic concept of children's welfare; second, the potential for developing civil rights for children through adult advocacy; and third, the scope for self-advocacy by young people.

Redefining child welfare

(The conception of welfare implied by the UN Convention incorporates the basic conditions children need for healthy development, including adequate income, housing, health, education and environmental issues: the conditions in which children might flourish)(CRDU 1994). This is not simply a broader agenda but also suggests the need for a corporate approach in organisational terms. While the early response of the UK government has not been encouraging, the Convention provisions do form the basis for a national policy strategy (CRO 1995) and are having some effect at the level of local strategy.

(Many issues of protection would be anticipated by properly addressing the basic conditions in which children might not just have an adequate standard of living but might actually flourish. The impact of poverty, its link with policies that reinforce state dependence for many families, the interrelationship between deprivation and risk to children's safety and well-being, and the higher risk of poverty for children from minority ethnic groups are well documented)(Cannan 1992; Segal 1995; Parton 1990; Kumar 1993; Oppenheim 1993).(Both direct and indirect forms of discrimination exist which structure children's experience according to their ethnic origin, gender or disability. Discrimination through racism, sexism or the absence of equality provisions in respect of disability, has particular consequences for children (in addition to those shared with adults) that can detrimentally affect their future welfare and autonomous adulthood)(Amin and Oppenheim 1992; CRDU 1994).(Overall, the impact of discrimination and poverty can be said to have a detrimental effect on human potential to assume full citizenship (Harris 1992). Furthermore, Rosenbaum (1993) has detailed the impact of environmental issues and pollution on children)

The model of child welfare on which policy in the UK is based is far narrower than this,)while concepts of the welfare or best interests of the child are absent entirely from much of the legislation affecting children's lives in the UK,(for example in respect of education, health and social security. Even in the Children Act 1989, the emphasis is placed on decision making in respect of the specific child within the family context, thereby limiting concerns about children's welfare to questions of individual need and protection from harm)(Boushel and Lebacq 1992; Smith 1991). The definition of need in the Children Act is based on a deficit model. The interpretation of need has therefore tended to be narrow and implementation hampered by a lack of resources (Boushel 1994; Bell 1993). Questions have been raised about one area of potential expansion – the inclusion of all children with disabilities in the category of children 'in need' under Section 17 of the Act – in the light of inadequate anti-discriminatory measures (Middleton 1995). Yet there is the potential in the Act for a broader preventive approach, which could contribute to the promotion of an environment in which all children may flourish (Smith 1995). Discussion of recent research (DoH 1995) concerning child protection and family support services seems likely to result in pressure towards an unhelpful bifurcation of the two rather than the required transformation in broader public policy relating to child need.

More positively, there are some signs, with the work on childrens' service plans by local authorities, of a more holistic and corporate approach to local policy in respect of children which is much more in line with the spirit of the UN Convention and with the obligations of the Children Act 1989 upon the local authority as a whole (AMA 1995).

Redefining welfare: young people's participation

I want to express my views on subjects I feel strongly about and hopefully do my bit to help.

(ROC Festival participant)

How can children contribute to the redefinition of welfare in this wider sense? Children have direct experience of the consequences of social policy, particularly in respect of education and the family, yet few opportunities to express views as young citizens. The diversity of their concerns suggests the need for a wide range of opportunities to participate. The provisions of Article 12 of the UN Convention clearly apply not just to the relatively narrow field of child care legislation but to 'all matters affecting the child'. As Freeman has pointed out, this is intended to include decisions in relation to the environment, education, transport, social security and so on, as well as to decisions within the family (Freeman 1993b).

The development of a young people's group called 'Article 12' represents a central element in an implementation strategy for the UN Convention, focusing on the active participation of children and young people in all levels of government, centrally and locally, and in all organisations (CRO 1995). A number of young people's forums already exist, representing diverse models of participation by young people in local decision making (British Youth Council – BYC). The key variations are their relationship with adult decision making processes; the extent to which they are led by young people; and their overall purpose – particularly whether this is primarily educative or concerned with empowerment.

One forum which represents the latter model is the Devon Youth Council. Youth council members provide the county council with young people's views, receive information on all 'significant issues' from all council departments and can raise issues with senior officers and committee chairs. In developing the role of the youth council, those involved recognised both the scepticism with which young people regard politicians and their commitment to pressure groups that link directly with their concerns.The adults have responded by 'analysing young people's resistances and activating them to become involved in their community as powerful agents for change' (Townsend and John forthcoming). Through outreach work the youth council has reached a wide group of young people and identified and acted on issues of concern to them, such as bullying. By co-ordinating work around regeneration for a 'rural challenge' bid, the youth council has demonstrated how young people can take a leading role in contributing to major joint initiatitives.

The Hove Schools' Council is a rather different forum, modelled on the local borough council although independent of it and with no direct say in that council's decisions. Its main objective is 'the education and development of understanding of the functions of local democracy among young people' (Hove Schools' Council 1991). Through the council, young people have taken the opportunity to undertake projects of particular concern to them, resulting in new facilities in the community and a drugs and smoking awareness campaign. Comments from young people involved included: 'It made me more aware, more responsible, better organised'; 'It has done a lot for me as a person'; 'It was education by getting out there and doing something'.

What young people seem to value most about such forums is the opportunity to influence decisions that affect them and the recognition that they are members of the community now as well as 'the decision-makers of the future' (East Cleveland Youth Council member).

Developing children's civil rights through adult advocacy

The CRDU *Agenda* (1994) details the range of civil rights issues that require attention in the UK for fulfilment of the UN Convention's requirements. These issues include civil liberties, physical integrity, nationality and immigration. While international law does not offer an accessible mechanism for relief in individual cases, the adoption of rights strategies at national and local level could enable individual claims to be addressed. Improving civil rights for children offers the prospect of better protection in a number of ways. The national strategy, proposed by the newly launched Children's Rights Office, spans a broad range of advocacy activities including the proposal for a Children's Rights Commissioner and the development of local children's rights officers (CRO 1995). These proposals, and others suggesting that 'child impact statements' be drawn up for all prospective policy developments, represent an attempt to address the current lack of priority accorded to children's issues in the political process and the lack of a voice for children (Rosenbaum and Newell 1991). Experience elsewhere suggests that such advocacy can raise the profile of children's interests and ensure effective means of complaint and redress (Flekkoy 1991).

The path towards recognition of children's legal rights to representation has been a chequered one. In England and Wales, the 1989 Children Act provides some opportunities for children to have their views heard in decision making, to make their own applications to the court in certain circumstances, to be represented and to have access to complaints procedures where local authority Social Services Departments are involved. However, there is a considerable disparity between children's rights in private, as against public, law proceedings. Children whose parents divorce have limited rights to have their views heard: if the care of children is uncontested, children are not able to express a view or object to the decision made and even, in contested proceedings, the child is not normally a party and will not be legally represented (CRDU 1994).[4]

The Gulbenkian report analyses the impact of negative attitudes to children together with the lack of a comprehensive policy towards child protection. 'We have all been conditioned by a culture in which deliberately hurting children is still accepted both socially and legally' (Gulbenkian Foundation 1993: xv). The report highlights the limitations of protective legislation and examines in particular children's lack of protection from violence in the home through the continued acceptance of physical punishment. The analysis suggests that protection will only be afforded by giving children direct rights of access to advocacy, representation and equal protection to that of adults under the law in respect of assault. Local advocacy services play an important role in enhancing access to existing measures of redress (e.g. Advice, Advocacy and Representation Service for Children – ASC). Beyond this, however, a higher priority needs to be accorded to the child's perspective. Boushel (1994), drawing on cross-cultural perspectives, suggests that the value accorded to children is a key factor in their protection, and that certain groups of children may be more vulnerable because they are less valued, whether by their families or the wider community.

Self-advocacy by children and young people

I liked it that I finally had a say in something that was important.
(ROC Festival participant)

Children have views concerning their own welfare and their own agenda of concerns: these are the two areas of interest referred to earlier. The following discussion draws on illustrations of activities in which children take the leading role in both these areas.

Young people who are 'looked after' by local authorities are likely to feel particularly powerless and isolated, not least as a result of discrimination which has been described as 'careism' (see NCC 1993; Ahmed 1993). Individual and collective self-advocacy approaches can help to reduce the stigma of such experiences. Many such forums for young people exist, facilitated by the local appointment of children's rights officers (CROA 1995) and some organisations are developing policies for children's rights with young people themselves.

The Upfront Support Team in Kent is one example of a group of young people with experience of having been in care who work with the children's rights worker to 'support and influence change for other young people who are looked after by the local authority' (personal communication 1995). They point to problems for individual children, for example in reviews:

> It is very difficult unless you are very confident and sometimes you don't have the same information as other people . . . so it's difficult to get taken seriously. They usually end up telling you what's in your best interests and you go along with it.

As a group they felt they could be heard and support young people's need for advocacy. The best things about the group were: 'having the chance to make a difference; meeting other people in a similar situation to yourself; feeling accepted; having the chance to discuss things.'

They also came up with 'Ten Commandments for Social Workers': qualities which they felt would make it easier for young people to be involved in decisions. Their number one rule was 'Never con yourself that you are the expert and NEVER EVER tell young people you know how they feel' (*Shout* 1995).

Both NAYPIC and Black and In Care had considerable success in representing young people in care on a national level during the 1980s. The latter survives together with groups which take their lead from young people, such as First Key, Voices from Care and the Who Cares? Trust. The Who Cares? north-east group of young people devised a description of a 'supportive adult'. This defines what young people mean by listening and respect, support and help and grew from discussions among young people about what they were seeking from the adults working with them. The qualities included: 'be committed to listening to and learning from young people'; 'be willing to check things out with young people'; 'be open'; and 'speak out in professional settings on behalf of young people'.

The group's statement includes rules on confidentiality and an agreed proviso on protection issues, demonstrating that negotiation on this was possible.

A rights perspective on child protection implies recognition and support of the child's potential for self-protection, acknowledging and maximising the strategies that children can use, while not placing sole reliance on them (Kitzinger 1990; Mullender and Morley 1994). While models of self-protection (e.g. Kidscape) should never divert attention from adult responsibilities in relation to abuse, there is much scope for the development of positive options for children, promoted by support services directly accessible to children (Saunders *et al.* 1995).

More generally, empowerment and participation for young people need to be set in a social context. Treseder (1995) emphasises that young people need to get something out of being involved in decision making and will seek fun and an addition to their social life and friendships, not just new skills. The emerging literature on involving children in the community emphasises the need for support, information and encouragement to young people with clear expectations and planned outcomes for all involved. Young people have little say in the provision of leisure activities and are heavily dependent on the goodwill of the adults who give up time to run local groups and clubs. The CRDU *Agenda* (1994) draws attention to the lack of a co-ordinated strategy for play and leisure, the impact of financial cutbacks, inequalities and discrimination in play provision and the lack of consultation with young people.

In their own evaluation of the success of the ROC Festival young people emphasised the importance of being able to determine the shape of the event and the nature of their participation in it from the start:

What was really good was getting to help organise it.
Usually there is an adult telling you you can't do something or checking up on you. We were given complete responsibility.

(ROC Festival participants)

It was important to the young people and adults involved that the emphasis on rights was implicit as well as explicit. Both the style and the content of the Festival were determined by the young people from the start of planning for the event, making the flavour of the day a fun one, and the whole process was led by young people and facilitated by adults. Comments from the younger participants demonstrated that a confident older teenager could disempower them as much as might an adult, indicating the need to facilitate mutual support and good models of empowerment between young people of different ages. The theme of rights was interpreted in a range of ways, providing opportunities for adults to listen to issues of importance to young people and to share in a celebration of their skills.

THE ROLE OF PROFESSIONALS IN PROMOTING STRATEGIES FOR CHILDREN'S RIGHTS

So far, it has been suggested that a children's rights perspective provides a framework for critically assessing current approaches to the protection of children, pointing towards strategies which assume a broader definition of welfare than child care professionals are currently encouraged to adopt and highlighting alternative forms of advocacy and self-advocacy that can assist children to participate in the definition of their own welfare. Two kinds of messages emerge: the first concerns the scope and orientation of social work with children and families while the second addresses questions about how professional workers might adopt a more participatory approach in their own practice.

Child protection and family support

In the current debate concerning the balance between family support and child protection little attention has been paid to a children's rights perspective (DoH 1995). Recent research has underlined the importance to child protection strategies of differentiation between family members (Farmer and Owen 1995) but the question remains as to how far models of family support that reflect these different needs will be forthcoming in the light of resource constraints. The challenge is to develop children's services plans into a comprehensive strategy, reflecting the broader definition of welfare discussed earlier and in line with the UN Convention.

The children's rights perspective suggests how work with children might be structured to maximise mutual support and self-advocacy, assisting them in conveying their own views concerning family difficulties both within the family and outside it and enabling them to feel more confident about their own claims. Young people need to feel that their needs are regarded as valid, that adults will respect them, that it is safe for them to raise personal issues and that the whole burden of family problems does not rest on their shoulders (Farmer and Owen 1995). This implies a re-orientation of work on 'parenting skills', ensuring consideration of respect for children's separate needs, discussion of practical alternatives towards rule making and discipline and addressing the operation of sexism in the family. The concept of 'dynamic self-determinism' could help to inform such work, suggesting as it does the developing nature of the child's ability to influence and make decisions. The UN Convention offers a perspective on 'positive parenting' within Article 5 and suggests the need to define 'parental responsibility' in a way which gives parents clear duties to promote their children's welfare and to do so in a manner 'consistent with the evolving capacities of the child' (CRDU 1994: 23).

Strategies should be emphasised which enable young people to support one another, whether through groups established for the purpose or through connecting young people 'in need' to local organisations which offer opportunities for self-development and different relationships with adults, thus providing a normalising experience for them.

Professional partnerships

Social workers and other professionals can explore links with rights and advocacy services and view positively the space they offer children to define their own needs and support. Young people may express a desire for complete confidentiality and this may conflict with the social worker's responsibility for protection. Yet it has proved possible for adults and young people to work together on such issues and reach solutions which feel safe and which enable young people to obtain support. The existence of independent support and advocacy, together with counselling and information services for young people, and self-advocacy groups can strengthen the available network of help for both young person and social worker.

The apparent decline of local, community-oriented approaches to the provision of social services, at least in England and Wales, reduces the likelihood of social workers having close contact with the local communities, schools and groups which structure the lives of the children and families with whom they work. Yet the opportunity presented by local corporate child care planning and strategies for youth, which offer a way forward for local implementation of the UN Convention, could assist social workers to renew their familiarity with other professionals and volunteers such as youth workers, advice workers, playleaders and community development workers.

Putting participation into practice

Young people have much to say about what they want from participation and about the adult behaviour that is most empowering, yet relatively little attention has been paid to their views. Some central issues in approaches to participation are indicated in the following two questions which both adults and young people can address at an early stage:

1   What is the purpose of the young people's involvement and is it agreed between adults and young people? For genuine participation, this must be negotiated at the outset. Adult encouragement for participation by young people may reflect a range of motives, which are not mutually exclusive. These may be tentatively characterised as follows: the 'future citizen' perspective, emphasising the educative potential of involvement and responsibility rather than rights; the 'consumer' emphasis, focusing on improving quality of provision and meeting expectations; the 'avoidance of exclusion', emphasising the consequences for the community of disaffected youth; and 'civil rights', linked with the redistribution of power towards young people. The notion of 'partnership' with young people in a child care context may reflect a number of these motives and the outcome in terms of participation will vary accordingly.

2   How can adults behave in a supportive and empowering way? The 'supportive adult' role to which we referred earlier needs to be worked on by adults and young people together in any given encounter and agreement reached on ways of reviewing how the distribution and balance of power is working. That young people value adults who will listen, guide and support them is clear from what they say: young people do not seem to want to take over the entire running of their own lives. 'Partnership' practice requires that the allocation of responsibility and power is negotiated between adults – both professionals and carers – and young people. This must be set in the context of need, risk and harm to young people which so shapes social workers' encounters with them. Above all young people need to know where they stand and what choices are open to them. Within organisations, an 'audit' of participatory practice should attend to the institutional structures and practices that inhibit children's involvement in decision making.

For young people to be enabled to take a lead role in developing their own interests and social concerns within a community context, adults must recognise children's competence and their 'project interests'. Youth forums will not be the preferred option for all young people, nor do all young people hold the same views. Support for young people's contribution is needed inside the organisations with which they are involved and a range of imaginative strategies is needed to enable young people to be heard. The approach of supporting young people with issues they have identified for themselves, as with environmental concerns, seems particularly successful (CRDU 1994; Children's Agenda 21 1994).

Some common threads

From the examples discussed in this chapter, several messages emerge which suggest a model for involving and listening to children:

- Young people value the opportunity to be involved in decision making, whether it affects only their own lives or those of a wider group, and they gain self-respect from such involvement. The opportunity to shape the agenda for involvement from the start is most highly valued.
- Through sharing experiences and working together, young people gain support from each other. Collective approaches can build on and develop friendship networks. However, it is essential to offer a wide range of opportunities for involvement, to reach a broad population of young people from all communities, to recognise the diversity of young people's interests and views and to attend to issues of age and gender.
- Young people want adult support and can offer guidelines as to the preferred form.
- Young people are particularly concerned about processes of communication and involvement, with issues of principle alongside questions of content. Unless the process is influenced by young people and shaped by their needs, adult attempts at encouraging participation will be unlikely to serve their stated purpose.
- When presented with such an opportunity, young people's contributions are often more imaginative than, as well as qualitatively different from, those of adults. There is much for adults to learn about service improvements from children.
- Young people's concerns cut across the divisions imposed by the adult world, just as the problems they face straddle the administrative categories of local and central government departments.

IN CONCLUSION

The above suggestions have been made in the recognition that social workers generally do their utmost to promote children's interests and take account of their views but that institutional as well as financial constraints often limit apparent opportunities to pursue alternative approaches. While it is essential for social workers to be aware of children's legal rights to have their voices heard in the context of domestic legislation, it is also important for staff within local authorities and voluntary organisations to contribute to the establishment of local strategies for implementing the UN Convention (for example AMA 1995).

Fundamental changes in attitude and strategies are needed for real-isation of the kind of child-friendly society envisioned by Newell (1995) and by the young people with whom we spoke. This will not come about simply through changes in individual practice but it can be furthered significantly by adults who understand children's own requests to be treated with respect and who can recall their own childhood longing to be heard.

The last word belongs to the young people:

Why shouldn't we be consulted about our future? Not only do these decisions concern us more than anyone else, I believe we also have a lot to offer and valuable opinions.

We have new and imaginative ideas.

We are the adults of tomorrow.

(ROC Festival participants)

NOTES

1 ROC 1995: The Young People's Festival of Rights took place in Brighton in July 1995. This event was the culmination of six months' work by young people and adults, with the dual aim of celebrating young people's talents and of providing young people with an opportunity to have their voices heard by politicians and other adults. The event built upon the work of a local group -- the Rights of Children and Young People Group (ROC) which aims to promote the UN Convention on the Rights of the Child. The quotes at the beginning of sections come from young people involved in the Festival and include some from members of VOYCE, a young people's environmental group.

2 The Children (Scotland) Act 1995 will, when implemented, give children such rights. This will incorporate Article 12 in primary legislation in respect of parents and other carers by giving the child the right to be consulted by them (Section 6). See Lansdown (1995).

3 The recent literature includes: representations of children's views on services and on problems (e.g. Butler and Williamson 1994; Farmer and Owen 1995; Saunders et al. 1995; NCH 1994; Dolphin Project 1993); practice principles for social work and community development in respect of listening to and involving children (e.g. Heaton and Sayer 1992; Butler and Williamson 1994; Cloke and Davies 1995); models, tools and techniques for participation and empowerment (e.g. Treseder 1995; Flekkoy 1991); discussion of the ethics of research with children (Alderson 1995); models of organising by and with young people (BYC; CRO).

4 Furthermore, in respect of consent to and refusal of medical treatment, while the 'Gillick principle' appeared to entitle a competent child to both,

subsequent court decisions have undermined this and mean that a child's refusal can be overridden (*Childright*, 115, April 1995, pp. 11–14).

REFERENCES

Ahmed, S. (1993) *Social Work with Black Children and their Families*, London: Batsford.

Alderson, P. (1995) *Listening to Children: Children, Ethics and Social Research*, Ilford: Barnado's.

Alston, P. (ed.) (1994) *The Best Interests of the Child*, Oxford: Clarendon Press.

Alston, P., Parker, S. and Seymour, J. (eds) (1992) *Children, Rights and the Law*, Oxford: Clarendon Press.

AMA (Association of Metropolitan Authorities) (1995) *Checklist for Children: Local Authorities and the UN Convention on the Rights of the Child*, London: AMA and CRO.

Amin, K. and Oppenheim, C. (1992) *Poverty in Black and White: Deprivation and Ethnic Minorities*, London: Child Poverty Action Group and Runnymede Trust.

Archard, D. (1993) *Children, Rights and Childhood*, London: Routledge.

Bell, V. (1993) 'Governing childhood: neo-liberalism and the law', *Economy and Society*, 22, 3: 391–405.

Boushel, M. (1994) 'The protective environment of children: towards a framework for anti-oppressive, cross-cultural and cross-national understanding', *British Journal of Social Work*, 24: 173–90.

Boushel, M. and Lebacq, M. (1992) 'Towards empowerment in child protection work', *Children and Society*, 6, 1: 38–50.

Butler, I. and Williamson, H. (1994) *Children Speak: Children, Trauma and Social Work*, Harlow: Longman.

BYC (British Youth Council) (n.d.) *Local Action: A Guide to Setting up a Local Youth Council*, London: BYC.

Carlen, P. and Wardhaugh, J. (1991) 'Locking up our daughters', in P. Carter, T. Jeffs and M. K. Smith (eds), *Social Work and Social Welfare Yearbook 3*, Milton Keynes: Open University Press.

Cannan, C. (1992) *Changing Families, Changing Welfare*, Hemel Hempstead: Harvester Wheatsheaf.

Children's Agenda 21 (1994) *Rescue Mission Planet Earth*, London: Kingfisher.

Cloke, C. and Davies, M. (eds) (1995) *Participation and Empowerment in Child Protection*, London: Pitman.

CRDU (Children's Rights Development Unit) (1994) *UK Agenda for Children*, London: CRDU.

CRO (Children's Rights Office) (1995) *Making the Convention Work for Children*, London: CRO (235 Shaftesbury Avenue, London WC2H 8EL).

CROA (Children's Rights Officers Association) (1995) *Directory of Children's Rights*, Coventry: CROA.

DoH (Department of Health) (1995) *Child Protection: Messages from Research*, London: HMSO.

Dolphin Project (1993) *Answering Back*, Southampton: CEDR, Department of Social Work Studies, University of Southampton.

Dworkin, G. (1971) 'Paternalism', in R. A. Wasserstrom (ed.), *Morality and the Law*, California: Wadsworth.

Eekelaar, J. (1986) 'The emergence of children's rights', *Oxford Journal of Legal Studies*, 6: 161.

—— (1992) 'The importance of thinking that children have rights', in P. Alston, S. Parker, J. Seymour (eds), *Children, Rights and the Law*, Oxford: Clarendon Press.

—— (1994) 'The interests of the child and the child's wishes: the role of dynamic self-determinism', in P. Alston (ed.), *The Best Interests of the Child*, Oxford: Clarendon Press.

Ennew, J. (1986) *The Sexual Exploitation of Children*, Cambridge: Polity Press.

Farmer, E. and Owen, M. (1995) *Child Protection Practice: Private Risks and Public Remedies*, London: HMSO.

Flekkoy, M. G. (1991) *A Voice for Children: Speaking Out as Their Ombudsman*, London: Jessica Kingsley.

Fox Harding, L. (1991) *Perspectives in Child Care Policy*, London: Longman.

Freeden, M. (1991) *Rights*, Buckingham: Open University Press.

Freeman, M. D. A. (1983) *The Rights and Wrongs of Children*, London: Frances Pinter.

—— (1992) 'The limits of children's rights', in M. Freeman and P. Veerman (eds), *The Ideologies of Children's Rights*, Dordrecht: Martinus Nijhoff.

—— (1993a) 'Laws, conventions and rights', *Children and Society*, 7,1: 37–48.

—— (1993b) 'Whither children: protection, participation, autonomy?' Conference paper, Institute for Public Policy Research.

Freeman, M. D. A. and Veerman, P. (eds) (1992) *The Ideologies of Children's Rights*, Netherlands: Martinus Nijhoff.

Frost, N. and Stein, M. (1989) *The Politics of Child Welfare*, Hemel Hempstead: Harvester Wheatsheaf.

Gulbenkian Foundation (1993) *One Scandal Too Many ... The Case for Comprehensive Protection for Children in all Settings*, London: Calouste Gulbenkian Foundation.

Harris, N. (1992) 'Youth, citizenship and welfare', *Journal of Social Welfare and Family Law*, 3: 174–92.

Heaton, K. and Sayer, J. (1992) *Community Development and Child Welfare*, London: Community Development Foundation.

Hodgson, D. (1994) Unpublished material from interviews with children.

Hove Schools' Council (1991) from the inaugural pamphlet, Hove Borough Council.

Kitzinger, J. (1990) 'Who are you kidding? Children, power and the struggle against sexual abuse', in A. James and A. Prout (eds), *Constructing and Reconstructing Childhood*, Basingstoke: Falmer Press.

Kumar, V. (1993) *Poverty and Inequality in the UK: The Effects on Children*, London: National Children's Bureau.

Lansdown, G. (1995) *Taking Part: Children's Participation in Decision Making*, London: IPPR.

McGoldrick, D. (1991) 'The United Nations Convention on the Rights of the Child', *International Journal of Law and the Family*, 5: 132–69.

McNay, M. (1992) 'Social work and power relations: towards a framework for an integrated practice', in M. Langan and L. Day (eds), *Women, Oppression and Social Work*, London: Routledge.

Melton, G. B. and Limber, S. P. (1992) 'What children's rights mean to children: children's own views', in M. Freeman and P. Veerman (eds), *The Ideologies of Children's Rights*, Dordrecht: Martinus Nijhoff.

Middleton, L. (1995) 'A disabling childhood', *Childright*, 113: 25–7.

Modi, P., Marks, C. and Wattley, R. (1995) 'From the margin to the centre: empowering the black child', in C. Cloke and M. Davies (eds), *Participation and Empowerment in Child Protection*, London: Pitman.

Mullender, A. and Morley, R. (1994) *Children Living with Domestic Violence*, London: Whiting & Birch.

NCC (National Consumer Council) and Who Cares? Trust (1993) *Not Just a Name*, London: NCC.

NCH Action for Children (1994) *The Hidden Victims, Children and Domestic Violence*, London: NCH.

Newell, P. (1995) 'Rights, participation and neighbourhoods', in P. Henderson (ed.), *Children and Communities*, London: Pluto.

Olsen, F. (1992) 'Children's rights: some feminist approaches to the United Nations Convention on the Rights of the Child', in P. Alston, S. Parker and J. Seymour (eds), *Children, Rights and the Law*, Oxford: Clarendon Press.

Oppenheim, C. (1993) *Poverty: The Facts*, London: Child Poverty Action Group.

Parton, N. (1990) 'Taking child abuse seriously', in *Taking Child Abuse Seriously*, Violence against Children Study Group, London: Unwin Hyman.

Perelberg, R. J. and Miller, A. C. (eds) (1990) *Gender and Power in Families*, London: Routledge.

Rosenbaum, M. (1993) *Children and the Environment*, London: National Children's Bureau.

Rosenbaum, M. and Newell, P. (1991) *Taking Children Seriously: A Proposal for a Children's Rights Commissioner*, London: Calouste Gulbenkian Foundation.

Saunders, A. with Epstein, C., Keep, G. and Debbonaire, T. (1995) *'It Hurts Me Too'. Children's Experiences of Domestic Violence and Refuge Life*, London: National Institute for Social Work.

Segal, L. (1995) 'Feminism and the family', in C. Burck and B. Speed (eds), *Gender, Power and Relationships*, London: Routledge.

Short, G. (1988) 'Children's grasp of controversial issues', in B. Carrington and B. Troyna (eds), *Children and Controversial Issues*, London: Falmer Press.

Shout (1995) Magazine of 'Upfront' Rights Service, Maidstone. May/June.

Smith, R. (1991) 'Child care: welfare, protection or rights?', *Journal of Social Welfare and Family Law*, 6: 469–81.

Smith, T. (1995) 'Children and young people – disadvantage, community and the Children Act 1989', in P. Henderson (ed.), *Children and Communities*, London: Pluto Press.

Townsend, P. and John, M. (forthcoming) 'Working towards the participation of children in decision making: a Devon case study', London: HMSO.

Treseder, P. (1995) 'Involving and empowering children and young people: overcoming the barriers', in C. Cloke and M. Davies (eds), *Participation and Empowerment in Child Protection*, London: Pitman.

—— (forthcoming) *How to Successfully Involve Children and Young People in Decision Making: A Training Pack for Participation and Empowerment*, London: Save the Children Fund/Children's Rights Office.

UNCRC (1989) *The Convention on the Rights of the Child*, United Nations. (Available from Children's Rights Office, London.)

Upfront Support Team (1995) Upfront Rights Service, Council for Social Responsibility, Canterbury and Rochester.

Wolfson, S. (1992) 'Children's rights: the theoretical underpinning of the "best interests of the child"', in M. Freeman and P. Veerman (eds), *The Ideologies of Children's Rights*, Dordrecht: Martinus Nijhoff.

Chapter 3

Mapping the future?

A contribution from community social work in the community care field

Peter Durrant

AN INTRODUCTION

This chapter aims to identify a range of contemporary practice examples which enable all of us to think more carefully about the style and nature of our intervention. Social work in the 1990s is in a poor state of health. Field, residential, day and support services have accepted a largely passive role, allowing crude top-down management structures to dictate the rules of the game. Grassroots practice has, to its discredit, generally colluded as local authorities and the independent sector have both moved too easily and even eagerly into naive purchaser–provider divisions. There has been little inclination for the thorough *and related* implementation of two major pieces of welfare law, the consequences of which have simply not been thought through. So the 1989 Children and the 1990 National Health Service and Community Care Acts are left somewhat in limbo.

What seems to be happening is that the *momentum* of change has effectively eliminated any discussion about the *rationale* of change. Social work, at a fragile time in its search for professional status, has been left adrift and vulnerable to attack by less well-established groups. This may well, however, be to its long-term advantage since unless we can think on our feet we have little to offer. Perhaps a more intelligent response is to understand what is happening historically and then, consciously and openly, to identify our values and strategies as a contribution to a fairer society. We could then tease out from our out-dated referral systems a more connected and operational way of working against the ever-present patterns of problems and, as Watts (1991: 215) has argued, follow 'in the tradition of Section 132 of the Social Work (Scotland) Act . . . in advocating a role for social work beyond that of client counselling and service provision'. Community social work recognises that the bulk of care, supervision and control in the community is undertaken by parents, neighbours, relatives, informal carers and other people operating through their normal social networks and amounts to 'a synthesis of individualised approaches to problems and community development activities' (Darvill and Smale 1990: 15).

SOCIAL SERVICES DEPARTMENTS AS THE MILLENNIUM NEARS

We clearly lack an overall sense of direction and, more seriously, we have only ourselves to blame for losing the way. Although there have been too many major organisational changes in the post-war years there have been a number of historical sign-posts at which we should, at the very least, have paused, and explored. These include the generic approaches following the Seebohm Report in 1968, community social work proposed by the 1982 Barclay Report and the underestimated Griffiths Report in 1988 on community care. This last built on the former reports in recommending a community social work approach to individual responsibility. Values that we should all more publicly debate.

While there seems good evidence that community social work, in Scotland at least, is alive and well, other unconsidered junctions seem to me to include the following:

(a) Considering whether social work is a trade or profession

Although both trade and profession reflect the acquisition of status, the former description, in terms of our personal and work status, is probably more useful. Whereas teaching, legal and medical career paths are sociologically well established, social work, to its credit, has sometimes been prepared to consider power, class and authority in relation to the usually vulnerable people who have most often been found to require its services.

Acquiring operational skills in the sense of social and community work as a trade has considerable advantages. It enables us to work more easily *with*, as opposed to *for*, people, to catalogue tasks together which need to be shared and, potentially, at least, sets the scene for evaluating completed work. Whilst elitist professionalism may be unable to relate clearly and warmly to people on the receiving ends of our complex systems, there *is* an interpretation of professional behaviour that is concerned with thoroughness, conscientiousness and public pain and poverty. What we should *not* be doing, which is what we *are* doing in the middle 1990s, is to collude with more influential and better placed policy makers' assertions that there is no need for a debate. But there *is* plenty of evidence that radical community development experiences are alive and well – although there is too little collective dialogue, without which we are all lost.

There are then distinct signs of creative and imaginative social and community work practice, even as children's and community care legislation, separately and unevenly, threatens to overwhelm us. Encouragingly, there are also indications emerging that more holistic alternatives *do* exist, although we all need to search for them more rigorously than we have previously been prepared to do. This chapter seeks to chart the nature of a different, but complementary, route for social and community work. The challenge for all in this decade is the same as it was in the 1980s: if, when and how we are prepared to tread these difficult paths . . .

(b) Exploring the usefulness of specialist and/or generic skill

The present divide which is widening daily between children's and adults' services illustrates this point sharply. Perhaps the argument is not about either/or situations but rather about how we should always remember that, unless we are prepared regularly to re-assess the route we have chosen, it is difficult to see how we can even begin our complex journey. We *must* have maps that include knowledge of political and social backgrounds, organisational cul-de-sacs and social policy indicators. We need an understanding of individual, group and community dynamics that would make it easier to comprehend how we all behave in situations of deep crisis. In this sense the concept of purchasing and providing, as an essential and always-present feature of power relationships, becomes a useful means of more accurately analysing transactions within and between people and agencies.

In other words, rather like the important work carried out in the 1980s by the National Institute of Social Work's Practice and Development Exchange, which worked outwards into the community from social work's existing practice base, it seems sensible not to reject the early social work traditions of understanding individual and group behaviours.[1] We also need to include more contemporary analogies with the market – commerce, the community and individual behaviour all need to be understood as a whole in the wider debate about social and community work at the turn of the century.

(c) Considering how our organisational styles affect our view of the world

Max Weber's analysis of, and distinction between, power and authority was, and perhaps is, the obvious starting point (Weber 1947). Local authorities, and this is increasingly true of the independent sector, do not systematise themselves by accident. Rather their middle and top management parts reflect the uneven ways in which society is structured. This has an especially dangerous effect as far as one-to-one, group and community work is concerned.

It means, for example, that practitioners too often feel they do not belong in the work of their employing organisation. Rarely are they encouraged to think about more reciprocal ways in which power can consciously be shared, how problem solving might become a corporate activity, and to question why large numbers of disadvantaged people *seem*, at various times in their lives, to *need* social workers.

(d) Action research and social auditing as a means of making sense of complex social situations

Remember Ronnie Laing as he struggled in the 1970s to understand double binds and other contradictory behaviours in complex family settings? In one short cameo (see Laing 1969: 17), he provides a good example of how social workers *always* find themselves in distressing, confusing dilemmas which usually seem unsolvable. His sharp awareness of how poor emotional health can destroy us all allows us to reflect on the histories of cultures, groups and nations, and to consider some of the alternatives. As he warns us, we 'must all continually learn to unlearn much we have learned, and to learn much that we have not been taught. Only thus do we and our subject grow' (ibid.).

Action research and the social auditing of our practice are commonsense ways of achieving this. These approaches help us all to set up an ongoing dialogue between the social scientist, fieldworker and organisations, including, as partners, peoples actually using services. Together, they make it possible to participate in identifying problems, formulating programmes and evaluating their effectiveness against other organisations and their goals. By locating and including a wider range of variables it then becomes possible to assess their effect on each other. 'It brings the client's understanding of his situation directly back to the agency concerned in the hope that services and communication could be improved at a local level' (Lees and Lees 1975: 171). Social auditing is a welcome contribution to turn-of-the-century evaluation strategies as a process that is systematic, comprehensive and regular; 'from the inside – assessing performance against its mission statement or statement of objectives; and, from the outside: using comparisons with other organisations' behaviour and social norms' (Zadek and Evans 1993: 3).

These four conceptual areas provide a starting point. As well as guidelines they are values; as such they represent real clues about how to proceed. After all if we are unsure why we are at the beginning of our professional expedition how can we possibly cope with the problems ahead? On the other hand if we have begun to think out our values stances, as well as our reasons for being there in the first place, strategies that could work can be more logically followed.

BUT WHY TRAVEL ANYWAY, OR ARE THERE ALTERNATIVE ROUTES?

Social work seems in this decade uncertain what direction to take. The British Association of Social Workers, increasingly failing to meet the needs of newer generations of social workers, is ambivalent about its ambition for a General Council backed up by a three-year qualification period, and critics see the new qualification, the Diploma in Social Work, as an attempt to meet government demands for more employer involvement in higher education and training and to prepare social work for greater regulation in practice (Cannan 1994–5). At the same time social services departments as purchasers find themselves hopelessly confused as they attempt to protect their existing in-house providers.

If would-be social workers accept the status quo only a dull form of professionalism awaits them. But there are alternatives. Social work courses themselves can, and should, be seen as an exciting and useful experience. As someone from a working-class background, I remember being heavily criticised by my middle-class colleagues when commenting on the privileges of education. Thirty years on, my opinion remains the same. We are fortunate people in an unequal world to have the opportunity to think and practise proactively and well.

These should be our golden years in which we creatively interweave and apply one social science perspective to another; shifting from the political and the psychological to sociology and links with social administration. And then, in spite of what that strange, but interdisciplinarily useful, term 'social work' means, to continue to argue and debate contemporary issues throughout one's lifetime.

Social work careers

These are an opportunity to meet and relate to people in need. Maybe at this point we should carefully consider some of the seductive uses of power and challenge the purpose of our over-protected reception areas and comfortable offices. There are few memories from my social work course on being streetwise and the importance of networking as an essential skill. But if we can learn these and other basic lessons early on perhaps they will stay with us as promotion prospects appear alluringly on the horizon.

Practitioners, of all varieties, have immense power and discretion. Not only do we have access to a wide range of support and administrative systems, telephones, faxes and, increasingly, the internet but we can also, if we choose, problem-solve within communities in creative and innovative ways. This is only possible if we have 'support' structures there to enable and facilitate change, not, as they often and more subtly do, to prevent it.

But what about our worker style?

One of the curious aspects of many social work courses and employer bodies is that they often seem to deny that we possess a wealth of life experience, pain and happiness to, potentially at least, share. Their, and our, response is, too often, that our own backgrounds have little or nothing to contribute when relating to others. Social work may be moving on from its over-ponderous case-work way of thinking about people as cases. Working on our worker style does not mean unwisely over empathising with people often in considerable distress, but it does mean finding the middle ground between the user's needs, the agency's dominance and a political view of the world. We always carry with us a great deal of political and psychological luggage and a failure to know what is in our professional suitcases means trouble. More optimistically if we have a fair idea of how we stand in relation to, say, poverty, unemployment, poor housing, exclusion and the like, the very stuff of social work, then we might make some progress.

This could be especially so as far as prevention is concerned. One of the worrying parts of social work education and practice today is that the concept seems to have disappeared without trace. Take this quote from a social worker writing to the *Guardian* in 1995 on Department of Health plans to reform child protection procedures by cutting the number of child abuse investigations. Commenting that the 'requirement to follow child protection procedures is an absolute imperative in every social work department' he notes that

> we operate the same procedures for a bruise as we do for major physical or sexual assault . . . hopefully the proposals will recommend that resources should be made available to families without their having to experience the humiliation of child protection procedures in order to just gain access to a service.[2]

What a good letter from a practitioner but why are there so few these days? We seem, strangely, unable to counter what he terms 'mechanistic and insensitive' processes' within public bodies.

This observation has been soundly backed up by Thorpe's (1994) evaluation of child protection which, a reviewer has argued, presents an analysis

> whereby images of child abuse and ever-widening definitions of abuse are used to establish new political ideologies of child protection. These serve covert purposes of social control and dominance of middle-class parents' norms; and withholding resources from parents who are struggling but who would succeed with appropriate services.

(Dale 1994: 29)

Nor are the dilemmas posed by work with people who are ageing and/or disabled any less relevant. Amongst the many issues community care and children's work have in common are people's crises and their pain within their problems. Both fields have opportunities to challenge the inevitability of situations which have occurred for generations, and to consider a means of exploring healthier alternatives in the future.

EXTENDING OUR WAYS OF WORKING: SOME EXAMPLES

What I am talking about is not just field, day, residential and support services but a broader definition of workloads and how we do our work. Although too many employing bodies, within and without the statutory sector, still have individualised referral systems there *are* different ways in which we can work more corporately. Changing one's style fundamentally influences the way one responds to the employing agencies. Think about it a little.

If we are prepared to argue that individual referrals have long histories prior to their points of crisis, then surely it makes sense to begin to think about their common elements. When children, families, individuals and communities find themselves in financial, housing, employment, legal and relationship difficulties and are then referred, by someone or other, to statutory and independent agencies, then is it not absurd if we ignore the problems which they share?

At this particular crossroad we all have choices. Do we continue to operate in ways that reinforce the agency's, our, *and* the consumer's, lack of power? Or do we begin to think about how resources might be better distributed? Are we really certain that problem definition and problem solving between different consumer groups are fundamentally different and therefore need to be handled differently? A few contemporary illustrations of how some people concerned with helping others to think about the causes of referred problems have thought about structural ways of operating, might help to make this point.

Prevention and children

If you are looking for departments prepared to take the lead, Kent social services is making a major shift in child care policy from investigation to prevention by creating eight nurseries in deprived areas.[3] Prevention is prevention is prevention as Gertrude Stein might have argued – whether you are 8 or 80.

We touched earlier upon the letter from a social worker arguing that the principle of prevention had lost too much ground to a sterile interpretation of child protection procedures. An Audit Commission report (1994), citing unpublished University of East Anglia research, suggested that up to two-thirds of cases of suspected child abuse are dropped before being considered for registration at case conferences.

But there are choices for us all. Newpin is a tangible demonstration of how people can be helped to behave in a different way, and to recover a sense of independence in immensely stressful situations. But you have to do something about the balance of power within organisations. This charity, based in South London but with several centres about the country, takes on mothers referred by health visitors, psychiatrists, social services and others. Women then relate to counsellors who befriend, support and advise them. But the crucial fact is that these counsellors are themselves formerly abusing mothers who are then used to support other mothers, who in turn may graduate to the same role.

At the top of this benign pyramid are professionals and the project works well because it enables women to help each other and fosters a cycle of self-respect, personal development, responsibility and true respect for others' individual rights. The children are being further helped by this network of peer support, despite the fact that many are on the child abuse register.[4] This is not dissimilar, perhaps, to the self-help initiative which began in the 1930s when people with drink problems began to work with each other through the group support of Alcoholics Anonymous. Newpin has never had a death or serious injury because, and perhaps here we are talking about applied common sense, it contracts with people to accept ownership of, and to do something progressive about, their own problems.

This is what the real transfer of power, as opposed to the fashionable concept of 'empowerment,' really means. It means networking in a positive and *skilled* way to problem-solve *in partnership with people*. Although our line management, and often absurd supervisory structures have a one-sided view of the world, we can alter our approach by shifting the goalposts. This what the London Borough of Haringey's specialist team did when providing intensive and specialist preventative work precisely for the purpose of reducing admissions to care. Recognising that bad housing, racism, unemployment and health issues played a role in families' struggles, their short-term focused intervention aims to keep children and young people in their communities, return them home where possible and ensure that where reception into care is in the child's best interest it is successful (Francis 1994).

There are one of two similar developments throughout the country which aim to provide round-the-clock help with people who are disabled or ageing. But these preventative messages too rarely find their way into neighbourhoods where isolated people could be helped to avoid 'three-o-clock in the morning' emergency admissions to institutional care.

Credit unions and community banks

These represent potentially radical ways of providing financial services to people under economic pressure. Many employer-led credit unions such as those in local authorities, the police and major industries have known this for years. But the statutory and independent sectors have failed, in the main, to consolidate the lessons which neighbourhood-based, inexpensive banking systems offer. Yet there may be ways forward as people debate and discuss some of the options that are beginning to appear in these last years of the century. One example is the Peckham Rye shop-front initiative which represents the second phase of credit union development initiatives in this country. Prior to 1993, most credit unions or community banks operated from small informal neighbourhood bases. This initiative, sponsored by the London Borough of Southwark, broke the mould by refurbishing a shop front and its employer-led credit union backs up the neighbourhood community bank. It now has 4,000 customers and over £2,000,000 managed in assets. Many people using the shop-front resource would, in all probability, not otherwise have been able to benefit from a cheap and supportive banking resource.[5] We know that in 1994 almost one in three children were living below the poverty line. We also know from the same source that the poorest tenth of the population suffered a 17 per cent fall in real income between 1979 and and 1992, after housing costs, and that their relative position continues to worsen (Department of Social Security 1994). Small sums of money from social workers and local authorities make little impact on these frightening statistics. Structural resources, as opposed to the divisive approach of much social work practice, would seem to be a better bet.

A second example is the Caerau Credit Union on the Ely estate in Cardiff which has begun to explore how debt redemption can be used to reach some of the most exploited and neglected members of an already impoverished community. It 'buys out' a person's, or family's, debts and then uses the credit union's low interest repayment rates of 1 per cent per month to manage their debts within a supportive community bank provision. The present transfer of money from the local authority, which has quickly seen its obvious benefits, is now over £10,000 per year. This confidence was reinforced by one customer for whom

> considering I didn't know about it in the first place it's brilliant. Something good is coming out of this. It's such a load off your head. Now I know there are other people in the same boat. I think it's brilliant.
>
> (Drakeford 1994: 9)

The potential of food co-ops

Remember that well-established community banks and foods co-ops can, quite legitimately, sponsor less fortunate communities to benefit from their profits and skills. This may be an important factor as National Lottery money begins to be allocated in 1995 for, initially at least, people and neighbourhoods in poverty and on low incomes. Examples are the Sandwell Food Cooperatives Development Unit in the West Midlands which supports seventeen community-run co-ops bringing cheap produce to more than a thousand local people and organisations (Moore 1995). Food co-ops are in their infancy. Could we do something to support them?

Health projects

The Ferguslie Community Health project in Strathclyde, with one of the highest unemployment rates in Scotland, has the philosophy of transforming victims into people taking some control over their lives. It leads to, as one of the organisers said, 'people labelled as failures at school or as bad mothers by social services [. . .] now running their own groups, talking at conferences and doing things they never imagined themselves doing'. One mothers' group tackled the estate's high child accident rates. The women, whose own children had suffered burns and other injuries in domestic accidents, recognised that local parents were no less caring than elsewhere. One problem was that they simply could not afford basic safety equipment. Since they launched a loan scheme for items like stair gates and fireguards, the number of child accidents treated at the local hospital has dropped (Moore 1995).

Well-organised urban community development initiatives

One well-known initiative of recent years is the work of the Phoenix Trust in Birmingham. Twenty years ago Balsall Heath presented a typical spectacle of inner-city decline with the manufacturing base of the area wiped out together with its community identity and spirit. Then a series of developments, led by local activists, brought about change through a nursery school being set up in the disused St Paul's Church Hall which included a care programme for families under pressure. In spite of the gangs of older children who regularly roamed and vandalised the neighbourhood, local people started an adventure playground. This grew into a purpose-built centre with a city farm, provided after-school clubs and eventually the St Paul's Community School, which is now registering more than encouraging results. Some of these children had not been to school for years. Now they leave with results that put much of the rest of the city to shame. One of the keys, as with all well-balanced community development work, is that children and their families see the school and other resources as an integral part of their local neighbourhood. Local people use it after hours since it 'belongs' to the community (Phillips 1993).

These brief introductions to community development themes are aimed at enabling social and community work practitioners, especially within local authority departments, to take a rounded view of the background of referrals and how they arrive on our desks. If we can learn to network proactively and publicly debate these issues then we have some chance of making a more effective contribution. A second look at worker style, for example, would suggest that if we read widely, especially newspapers and government documentation, and scan media sources intelligently we would soon accumulate a range of ideas and suggestions that would move us on. We could then, as a professional statement of intent, build data-collection time into our workloads, and start action research and social audits of these issues.

The point here is that unless we take an eclectic view of our work, are prepared to stay regularly close to practice, and encourage ourselves and our agencies to think and debate issues as they are happening, we will not have moved our trade on. There are no easy answers but if we can (and this is an old social case-work principle) start from where children, families and individuals are at, then we will at least have a few clues about how to proceed. Look at the evidence that surrounds us. The Urban Community Network, which has sixty centres in the most deprived areas of Britain's cities, manages 1,000 different projects which are used by 100,000 people per week. Their evidence is that 'where individuals are linked with "Second Chance to Learn" schemes over seventy per cent find either a job or a full-time place on a further education course' (Matthews 1994). Eastham's community social work in Canklow, based in a family centre, found a large decline over two years of children on the at risk register (Eastham 1990). In Oldham, Rogowski (1993) reports that community social work led to an increase in informal callers but a dramatic 85 per cent drop in official referrals. Again, Gibbons's analysis of neighbourhood family centres found them adept at attracting needy families and at involving them in community activities (Holman 1993). These three studies are from an article in the *Guardian* by Bob Holman, who, before he become a community worker on Glasgow's Easterhouse estate, held the Chair in Social Administration at Bath University. One of Bob's many strengths is that he applies his academic knowledge to grassroots practice situations in the national press. With tremendous effect.

The proof is not difficult to find if we are prepared to apply the academic evidence and theories we learn to the life experiences we collect informally, using them constructively to question the status quo and especially our own practice. One present organisational barrier to this is that the separate community care and children's legislation are effectively creating two different departments within social services. We should remind our employers, and ourselves, that a White Paper (Department of Health 1989: 3) argued that 'the two programmes are consistent and complementary and, taken together, set a fresh agenda and new challenges for social services authorities in the next decade'.

What actually followed in the early 1990s was an obsession with fashionable and untried management techniques which overwhelmed discussion on the proven usefulness of collaborative notions of partnership, which, in many people's experience, actually works. There is nothing wrong in buying services and resources from reputable and creative sources, as long as it is part of an interrelated exercise and we fully involve the customers in the transactions.

MAPPING THE FIELD: WAYS FORWARD IN THE 1990S

This last section examines some general ideas founded on community work principles of a shared and open debate, grassroots-upwards practice and a commitment to intelligent networking. Community social work is about extending individualised referrals to a collective view of problems which, in many situations, possess the same root causes. A common view is that child care, often from within family and drop-in centres, has dominated our thinking (as indeed it should), but we should not deny a generic view of communities. After all, life for all of us is a plural and shared experience. We all live and die, are members of families, encounter a range of painful and satisfying experiences throughout our existence and live in some sort of integrated setting.

The ideas that follow are offered as a means of identifying reciprocal styles of work which enable all of us to debate social action within social and community work with children and families. They are styles that also work well with people with a range of disabilities and with the rest of us who are ageing.

1 *Brokerage approaches*. There is no one specific model but this is a common theme in good social and community work practice. Through being an independent adviser, preferably one step removed from your employing body, you can quickly and effectively identify a wider range of alternatives. It ties in with working with customers who have control of their own budgets, but who can also work skilfully on testing pragmatic advice on how and when one sensitively in-fills. It is a model, as Steve Dowson has argued, that has little in common with the limitations of care management, making it really worth a second look.[6]

2 *Community businesses and social firms* can offer more inclusive opportunities for disabled, disadvantaged and unemployed people to change direction. Scotland, for various reasons, is well ahead of the rest of the country although East Anglia is emerging well with community

enterprises focusing on niche open-market trading areas such as organic farming, wooden sculpting, ceramics and furniture design, tea rooms and cafés, recycling schemes, community print opportunities, print-finishing and a mustard factory.[7]

3   Young people from the Broxtowe estate in Nottingham, fed up with hanging around the community centre, came up with the idea of setting up their own businesses. The venture failed, but Broxtowe Estate Enterprises rose from the ashes to provide a range of community options. For those on the estate, as well as for thousands of others in disadvantaged areas around Britain, community businesses offer do-it-yourself re-generation, from community shops and launderettes to credit unions and housing co-operatives. If you really work on alternatives, look at the Hulme estate in Manchester, where new developments are incorporating flats owned by the community as a housing co-operative with 20,000 square feet of community works space. These two projects describe some of the many community businesses 'which could make Labour's public ownership debate irrelevant to many' (Cowe 1995). In many social services departments the business ethic is already with us, and perhaps, if we can point it in a more socially aware direction, it has a great deal to offer.

4   One way of demonstrating this approach may well be through the potential community benefits of local exchange trading schemes, which are developing more targeted ways of helping people on low incomes as they break away from more middle-class bartering systems. The Beck-ford Mental Health Team in Warminster[8] is currently offering a project that enables residents experiencing depression and other mental health problems to help themselves and others in a similar situation. It also has a range of drop-in groups, sponsored walks and complementary therapies from acupuncture to reflexology. Could LETS options encourage and reinforce reciprocal relationships and move on to work with disad-vantaged children and families?

5   *Working professionally and politically with neighbourhoods.* There is considerable evidence that party politics and democracy are not synonymous. Try measuring this statement by asking yourself how close councillors are to our operational notions of aetiology and practice. It seems obvious that we should be constantly re-examining more particip-ative models of local government as part of our professional respons-ibility of involving people on the margin in order to make more use of mainstream services. One good example involves the extension of tenant power, a central element of Hackney's Comprehensive Estates Initiative, which is aimed at regenerating five of Hackney's more ravaged local

estates. Women in various circumstances are central to the success of the project, which provides for mothers with young children – single parents or otherwise – to re-enter the job market (Hill 1995).

6 *Borrowing national and international ideas.* In 1995, prior to moving on to a professorship at Keele University, Jane Tunstill set up a data bank at the University of East Anglia called the Family Support Network which aims to provide advice and research on family support services. Florida's Last Chance Ranch sounds the last place to achieve results within juvenile justice systems but its more liberal approach, which moves radically away from 'boot camps' and other autocratic regimes, seems promising. The style is based on character-building, outward bound-style activities with firm discipline and the forging of close relationships between staff and students. Fewer than four in ten teenagers, and we are talking about young people who are only sent there when Florida's youth justice schemes have given up trying to deal with them, get into trouble within three years of finishing the eighteen-month programme (Katz 1992). In Roubaix, France, 620 two-year, on-the-job training places in centres were created, with half the young people coming from one-parent families, often from households where the parents are also out of work. These were employment alternatives for the growing army of people excluded from the labour market (Steel 1994). The 1978 closure of psychiatric hospitals in Pordorene in Italy has led to *integrated co-operatives*, or *social enterprises*, employing 500 men and women with mental health problems in sanitation, welfare and gardening occupations.[9]

7 *Rethinking the 1982 Barclay Report.* Six years after the publication of the Barclay Report, Roy Griffiths built upon its recommendations by emphasising a community approach to individual problems, with a closer relationship between a variety of agencies, and a greater involvement of consumers, carers and their families in decision making about what services are provided at what times and in what ways. These strategies apply equally to families, to children with special needs and to more obviously disadvantaged youngsters.

8 Anne Williams (assistant director with 'Action for Children in Wales') in her study of the *users of two family centres* showed how they negotiated, within the purchaser–provider split, new working relationships with social services departments. The Parents Committee at Llanedeyrn produced a list of seventeen requirements, including that of social workers not outnumbering parents at meetings, and that professionals should listen to what users have to say. Its parallel in Crediton

demonstrated evidence of successful work based on a clear provider role, control over resources, access to money, more independence and a stronger bargaining position (Dobson 1994).

9   *Thinking in more inter-disciplinary ways* with schools and other community resources who are prepared to innovate. St Anne's primary school is just a hundred yards from where the Toxteth riots began in an area of unemployment, broken homes, drugs, prostitution and joy-riding. But in the early 1980s the school launched an experimental centre which turned people's lives round. It helped parents to become involved, developed workshops to relieve tension and encourage a sense of control with 'the idea that this generation of parents can be doers instead of victims' (Houghton 1995). Neighbourhood crime is down and the borrowing of library books is up.

10   *Turning the problem upside down.* If creative social and community approaches involve social enterprise, ownership and participation then perhaps self-build could be the answer. The Children's Society is working on projects for young people in housing need and leaving care; nine young people are building their own homes. They receive a lump sum in return for their labour on the scheme and can then rent on completion (Holman and Gillon 1994).

11   *Investing in potentially important developments.* Whether or not we get a Labour government in the late 1990s the Commission on Social Justice (1994) contains a number of interesting leads on how to move community services on. One option is community development trusts in 250 disadvantaged areas supported by a National Community Regeneration Agency.

12   *Although do beware the myth of the hero innovator.* An essay that should be read and re-read, throughout our professional lives, nicely challenges

> the idea that you can produce, by training a knight in shining armour who, loins girded with new technology and beliefs, will assault his organisational fortress and institute changes both in himself and others at a stroke. Such a view is ingenuous. The fact of the matter is that organisations such as schools and hospitals (*and they could easily have included social services departments*) eat hero innovators for breakfast.
>
> (Georgiades and Phillimore n.d.: 2; emphasis added)

Organisational guidelines *do* exist which enable us all to avoid such a dreadful fate.

And so one could carry on. All around us through developing media opportunities, literature, politics and the new information highway (Durrant 1995) there is a wealth of options which can help us to measure both how we professionally perform and how we might then reappraise our journeys. We can take a more inclusive, inter-disciplinary route, *with* our customers, as we proceed. We should also remember our European destiny. Just as the original objective was to try and prevent the possibility of yet another continental war so, too, there are growing numbers of international opportunities between Brussels and the rest of the world waiting to be explored.

Let's travel together . . .

NOTES

As this chapter argues we are all social and community work salesmen, with inquisitive toes in other people's doors. What follows is a variety of leads which might help to make for more satisfied customers.

1 Building upon the work of the *Barclay Report*, Barbara Hearn, Gerry Smale and others made the most of their Rowntree Trust finance to break new ground, leaving us with half-a-dozen seminal books from the National Institute for Social Work, Mary Ward House, 5–7 Tavistock Place, London WC1H 9SS.

2 Letter to the *Guardian* 5/6/93 by a Cambridge social worker, Vince Hesketh, who, to the astonishment of management, and the appreciation of field-workers has consciously remained a practitioner now for almost twenty years.

3 'Kent shifts to prevention.' News item in *Community Care*, 20 April 1995.

4 It is unusual to include people actually involved in child abuse situations to use their experience to help others, but you can find out more from National Newpin, Sutherland House, 35 Sutherland Square, London SW17 3EE.

5 You can find out more about the shop-front credit union at 221 Rye Lane, Peckham, London SE15 4TP. The Caerau Credit Union is located on the Ely estate in Cardiff.

6 David and Althea Brandon have written a great deal about brokerage concepts and their publications can be obtained from 50 Regatta Ct, Oyster Row, Cambridge CB5 8NS. Steve Dowson, former Director of Values into Action, is the author of the booklet, *A Review of the Service Brokerage Model in Community Care*. This makes some interesting comparisons between care co-ordination, social work and brokerage strategies. Available from VIA, Oxford House, Derbyshire St, London E2 6HG.

7 Try Peter Durrant on 01223 262759 for a discussion about some East Anglian community enterprises.

8 Try Beckford Community Health, The Beckford Centre, Gypsy Lane, Warminister, Wiltshire.

9 See 'Co-operation as a social enterprise in Italy; a place for social integration and rehabilitation.' Published in Italy but copies are available from Peter Durrant on the telephone number above. Or e-mail: thedurrants@cityscape.co.uk

REFERENCES

Audit Commission Report (1994) *Seen But Not Heard – Executive Summary*, London: HMSO.

Barclay Report (1982) *Social Workers: Their Role and Tasks. The Report of a Working Party*, London: National Institute for Social Work.

Cannan, C. (1994–5) 'Enterprise culture, professional socialisation and social work and social work education in Britain', in *Critical Social Policy*, 14 (3): 5–18.

Commission on Social Justice (1994) *Social Justice: Strategies for National Renewal*, London: Vintage.

Cowe, R. (1995) 'Solutions that lie with people', *Guardian*, 25 April.

Dale, P. (1994) 'Dangers in abuse's new ideology', *Community Care*, 15–21 September.

Darvill, G. and Smale, G. (1990) *Partners in Empowerment: Networks of Innovations in Social Work*, London: National Institute for Social Work.

Department of Health (1989) *Caring for People: Community Care in the Next Decade and Beyond*, presented to Parliament by the Secretaries of State for Health, Social Security (CM 849) London: HMSO.

Department of Social Security (1994) *Households Below Average Income*, London: HMSO.

Dobson, R. (1994) 'Attainable goals', *Community Care*, 10–16 November.

Drakeford, M. (1994) 'Credit unions and debt redemption', *Social Action*, 2 (2): 4–10.

Durrant, P. (1995). 'A world in your web', *Guardian*, 19 April.

Eastham, D. (1990) 'Plan it or suck it and see', in G. Darvill and G. Smale, (eds), *Partners in Empowerment: Networks of Innovations in Social Work*, London: National Institute for Social Work.

Francis, J. (1994) 'Home work', *Community Care*, 10–16 March.

Georgiades, J. N. and Phillimore, L. (n.d.) 'The myth of the hero-innovator and alternative strategies for organisational change.' Department of Occupational Psychology, Birkbeck College, University of London.

Gibbons, J. (ed.) (1992) *The Children Act 1989 and Family Support: Principles into Practice*, London: HMSO.

Gibbons, J., Thorpe, S. and Wilkinson, P. (1990) *Family Support and Prevention. Studies in Local Areas*, London: HMSO.

Griffiths, R. (1988) *Community Care: Agenda for Action. A Report of a Working Party*, Department of Health, London: HMSO.

Hill, D. (1995) 'Towering agenda gets real', *Guardian*, 25 March.

Holman, B. (1993) 'Pulling together', *Guardian*, 20 January.

Holman, B. (1994) 'Ethics, strength and values', *Community Care*, 10–16 November.

Holman, C. and Gillon, P. (1994) *Making Community Self-Build Happen*. London: The Children's Society.

Houghton, B. (1995) 'Back to school for success', *Guardian*, 21 December.

Katz, I. (1992) 'Velvet glove is mightier than the boot for Florida's teen tearaways', *Guardian*, 3 June.

Laing, R. D. (1969) *Intervention in Social Situations*, London: Association of Family Caseworkers and the Philadelphia Association.

Lees, R. and Lees, S. (1975) 'Social science in social work practice. The case for an action-research approach', *British Journal of Social Work*, 5 (2): 161–74.

Matthews, J. (1994) Letter in *Guardian*, 6 September.

Moore, W. (1995) 'A hundred ways to healthy living', *Guardian*, 20 April.

Phillips, M. (1993) 'The wonderful world of people's power', *Observer*, 5 December.

Phillips, M. (1994) 'Social work that can actually work', *Guardian*, 18 December.

Rogowski, S. (1993) 'Community social work with children and families: a positive step forward', *Journal of Applied Community Studies*, 1 (3): 4–22.

Seebohm Report (1968) *Committee on Local Authority and Allied Personal Social Services* (Cmnd 3703), London: HMSO.

Steel, J. (1994) 'French show sensitivity to the plight of the shut outs', *Guardian*, 29 July.

Thorpe, D. (1994) *Evaluating Child Protection*, Milton Keynes: Open University Press.

Watts, S. (1991) 'Community social work', in Lishman. J. (ed.), *Handbook of Theory for Practice Teachers in Social Work*, London: Jessica Kingsley.

Weber, M. (1947) *The Theory of Social and Economic Organisation*, Glencoe: Free Press.

Zadek, S. and Evans, R. (1993) *Auditing the Market. A Practical Approach to Social Auditing*, London: Traidcraft Exchange and New Economics Foundation.

Chapter 4

Social development with children and families in France

Crescy Cannan

INTRODUCTION

In this chapter I want to describe some of the changes which have been occurring in the social welfare field in France. The significant feature of contemporary French policy is the integration of social planning, around the goals of preventing exclusion and of promoting integration (or *insertion*), across a wide range of services, agencies, professions and community groups. This means that in the case of families, children and youth we immediately find we are looking at 'territorialised' strategies which include not only labour market measures but community development initiatives, usually referred to in France as local, or urban, social development. There have been enormous implications for the social work professions.

France makes an interesting comparison with the UK because in both countries there have been rigorous attempts to confront the issue of the cost of welfare states, and a search for new means of promoting as well as delivering social welfare. In the 1980s France's social democratic governments tackled issues of welfare dependency with an emphasis on the responsibilities of both state and citizen in the development of personal welfare and social cohesion. The election of a right-wing government in the early 1990s has not fundamentally challenged this; the long tradition of republicanism and Catholicism means that one-nation Gaullism continues to assert the importance of 'society' (*le social*), though it might be more willing to implement cuts in welfare expenditure to reduce budget deficits, and to ignore the social partners in so doing (Silver 1994).

My information comes from observation visits over six years to a *département* in north-west France where I have come to know social welfare practitioners, managers, social work trainers and sociologists.

What I hope to convey in this chapter is a picture of the innovations in social provision and practice, as well as the things that are proving problematic for the social welfare professions and for those who use (or might use) services. I will let the French speak directly, drawing from taped interviews carried out in the summer of 1995, and discuss the policy and intellectual framework of contemporary social development strategies in relation to children and families, stressing the distinctive feature (for British observers) of French social policy – a sociological perspective, a stress on the obligations as much as the rights of citizenship, a focus on promoting participation and conviviality in the public sphere, and the development of innovative and flexible forms of service in meeting contemporary needs.

THE CONTEXT OF FRENCH SOCIAL ACTION: URBAN SOCIAL DEVELOPMENT AND NEW LOCAL POWERS

Public administration in France began a process of modernisation under Mitterrand, the Socialist President, from the early 1980s. Decentralisation was intended to re-orient professionals to local social and economic conditions, to break the hold of traditional administrative norms, and to encourage strategic thinking. The welfare state was already perceived as entering a crisis of costs and as being outmoded in its attitudes to users. It was seen to be promoting passivity and dependence as well as failing to meet the contemporary needs of citizens. There followed an ambitious set of programmes to promote the social and professional *insertion* of youth and the long-term unemployed, to prevent delinquency and to promote regional economic development. A major programme was the *Développement Social des Quartiers* (DSQ), which like the others rests in commissions in which strategy is planned, implemented and evaluated 'transversally', across departments and agencies (see Cannan (1995) for a fuller account of the DSQ programme, in which 400 schemes were operating in the early 1990s). The interministerial *Delégations* and *Directions* at national level complement interagency commissions at local level. Budgets from separate departments are spent on common programmes, the whole currently being co-ordinated by contracts that the state makes with the cities or regions. These *Contrats de Ville* expect that, at the local level, planning is appropriate to local conditions and needs and yet reflects the big national principles – *insertion*, prevention of exclusion, economic and social development, partnership. By 1993, 185 contracts had been approved (Le Galès and Mawson 1994).

Social action in France means the practical application of social policy; it includes social welfare services for the protection of children and the promotion of families *and* associated family benefits. It is a shifting, diverse field, especially at present when the decentralisation process continues to throw up new centres and relations of power. This means that welfare services can be found in the social services of the *département* (equivalent to a county), in independent welfare organisations contracted to carry out particular elements of social policy, and in the most significant insurance fund in social action terms, the Caisse Nationale d'Allocations Familiales and its decentralised organisations, the Caisses d'Allocations Familiales (CAF) of individual *départements*. This is the principal family benefits organisation; a private organisation, it is nevertheless regulated by government policies on benefits and their levels. Local contracting and contracts between state and city produce a diversity of arrangements combined with coherence in objectives and principles because these are enshrined in five-yearly National Plans.

Decentralisation gave the responsibility for social action and certain public health services to the *départements*. What is currently complicating the picture is that the cities (and their communes) are becoming powerful providers and promoters of local social development. The social sphere, or social action, used to be a sleepy and dull backwater, but now it's everyone's business:

> it's true that the more the city intervenes at the social level, notably because of the economic and employment crisis, the urban becomes a decisive, strategic place for policy and the cities have understood that. Urban policies are becoming more and more difficult with the closure of businesses and factories and the problems of the *banlieues* [large outlying estates]. Conflict is moving from the workplace, the factory into the urban space, the neighbourhood. So more and more people are saying social work is my business. . . . Social action is . . . the policy not just of intervention on the ground, but the use of a certain number of funds for leading a certain number of policies.
>
> (M. Cardi, sociologist and manager in a family welfare agency)

There is then a new local interest in the management of the crisis, an interest shared between elected local politicians (*élus*) and those in the social field who manage it. Housing (and social housing is a significant field in France), health, youth, social services and schools have a stake in the prevention of local social decline. But because the *départements* have responsibility for social action there are complex relations with the cities and their communes:

> In relation to the actions of the commune, *département* and CAF it's not quite competition, but it's not simple . . . things were mostly moved from the State to the *département*, to be closer to citizens. . . . So there has been for several years reflection at the national level on the ways of organising social action in the *départements*. Not all *départements* have advanced in the same way or at the same pace, [but] . . . it has begun a preoccupation with the organisation of social action. . . . The commune doesn't really have a place, it's a subject of debate, but I think it will happen quickly because of the multiplicity of centres of decisions in social action such that one doesn't know who does what. . . . On the ground there are professionals who belong to the commune, to the CAF, *département* and more from associations which have agreements with the *département*, so it's not always well coordinated. . . . So we are in a phase where we have to consider a more simple organisation of social action on the ground.
>
> (M. Naveau, social worker and director of commune's social action centre)

Not surprisingly there is conflict:

> Social problems are not necessarily more easy to manage where more and more people are involved with them. . . . Today there is almost a quarrel over legitimacy – between the technical legitimacy of professionals and the political legitimacy of the *Conseil Général* [the County Council].
>
> (M. Troussier, sociologist who teaches in a social work college)

A PORTRAIT OF SOCIAL ACTION FOR CHILDREN AND FAMILIES

Services for children and families are situated in this context. The trends within the field are familiar: rising anxiety about and mounting referrals concerning child abuse, a trend away from using children's homes and a development of fostering and more flexible arrangements designed to help children and young people remain at home (Corbillon 1993). What are more specific to France are the very high levels of day care provision for children and the continuing expansion of nursery schooling from age 3. Much is politically invested in this popular, generous system of services which is being adapted to changing and more rigorous economic circumstances by, for instance, looking at more flexible use of child care resources, and the use of foster parents, child minders and parent-run crèches alongside institutional provision. Because the health and welfare systems are running in deficit there is an urgency behind this search for innovative family support measures.

For children and youth, policy continues to emphasise participation in the public sphere, referred to as *socialisation*; this is seen as necessary for children of all social classes and it complements schooling, significantly an area of social policy that remains centralised. Combined with the concern to prevent delinquency, which is understood as a crisis of employment and a lack of appropriate training, the whole of social action for children and youth can be seen as focused on *insertion sociale et professionnelle* (social and employment integration) and thus on the overall goal of solidarity.

How does the jigsaw fit together on the ground? An example is the city we shall call 'Ville', whose three main children and families services are the Centre Socio-Culturel (run by CAF), the Circonscription d'Action Sociale (an area office with social and health workers from the *département*'s social services), and the city's Centre Communal d'Action Sociale. There are also several well-resourced municipal crèches and youth centres. Because this is a very dynamic city the co-ordination between these organisations is good, though it takes a lot of energy to work in this framework. The city needs it: as a new city built in the boom years of the 1960s, it now faces a collapse of employment, it has a heterogeneous population with many ethnic groups, and families with great difficulties. Nevertheless the spirit is one of optimism; people still want to come and live in the city which is well tended and landscaped; its housing services are extensive and imaginative (and have a history of housing renovation and community development schemes such as *Habitat et Vie Sociale* from the 1970s) so that the blocks of flats are softened, reminding one of the original aspirations that such cities could be places of hope rather than isolation and vandalism.

The Caisse d'Allocations Familiales: socio-cultural centres for families and children

CAF provides social action as a separate but complementary service to its benefits (it provides varied levels of social action in different *départements* according to local contracts). In our *département* it provides a network of socio-cultural centres, which are well-resourced family and community centres offering flexible day care for children.

The centres also have social work services, maternal and infant health care provided by the *département*, health visitors, *conseilleurs en economie sociale et familiale* (CESF) who provide group activities on family life and home building in the context of housing as well as the management of benefits, and *animation socio-culturel* – leisure activities. The social work service shares, under convention, some of the statutory work in relation to child protection with the social workers of the *département*.

CNAF's main priorities for social action for 1992–6 are to offer services to families which complement family benefits. These services are in the main day care services for children which are offered through *contrats enfance* with the *département*, leisure activities to support families in their everyday life, and help for families in difficulties. It is clearly stated that these services should not be substituted for those already in place in the local health, cultural, leisure, etc. spheres, and that CAF works in partnership with local organisations in order to gain the greatest possibility of innovative and locally relevant social action. A global policy is always an objective: families are supported across the sectors of their working, domestic and school lives, and child care services are being made more flexible in order to meet current realities of family and working life (CNAF 1992). CAF social centres contribute to the life of families and to the social life of the neighbourhood: they are firmly within the overall French approach of social development and *action globale* – locally rooted, multi-agency, generic action for solidarity.

The CAF centre in 'Ville' fulfils its mission as follows:

> For me the crèches are prevention as well as promotion. . . . We are adapting to the changes in the family, for instance the *halte garderie* (nursery) has completely changed its timetable, it offers different patterns of care, for instance by the hour, by the half day, or for the whole day because there are lots of women who are looking for work or courses and have to start at once so they can say yes, no problem. . . . Child care is still principally for the socialisation of children, prevention of abuse is secondary.
>
> (Mme Ledoux, CAF child care adviser)

While its social workers and health visitors will have individual child protection cases, they are also required to work collectively, with schools, youth workers and perhaps with the *animateurs* and CESFs to devise ways of promoting mothers' confidence and of reducing their isolation. The centre has excellent workshops for its activities and courses in pottery, silkscreen printing and so on and seeks to maximise community use of these. There have been projects, for instance, of working together with residents to decorate the entrances and staircases of blocks of flats, and the centre seeks continually to adapt its activities to help parents with the practicalities of maintaining their flats, of managing on small incomes, and of providing a good diet. There have been projects with the local primary school – *Parlons Ensemble* (let's talk together) and *Ateliers de Langage* (language workshops) which help parents to understand the expectations of schools and show them how they can affect their children's progress. The emphasis on shared leisure is strong, with groups of parents and young people (perhaps with local youth workers) working together on activities that enable them to plan and then go on holiday or summer outings together (*Loisirs Familiaux de Proximité* and *Pause Café*).

This approach to supporting families through the flexible use of a centre's resources will be familiar to anyone working in a good family or community centre in Britain. What is distinct in the French context is the breadth of co-ordination between agencies and local government projects and a sense of longer-term partnership and planning. This is beginning to happen across the care/education divide for young children, because nursery schooling (along with child minding) is being promoted as a cheaper alternative to crèches. Because nursery school classes are large CNAF opposes them as a form of care but will support policies if there is a child care professional alongside the teacher:

> CNAF is funding *éducatrices de jeunes enfants* [qualified child care workers] to work in nursery schools; . . . CNAF does not want to finance schooling, but it helps disadvantaged families with young children go to school at 2. The primary school teacher . . . can be alone with twenty-five, even in some *départements*, thirty-two. . . . So in education priority areas, where the children are admitted at 2 (though it's 3 normally), CNAF has started to finance care of children in schools on condition they hire a child care worker.
>
> (Mme Ledoux, CAF child care adviser)

There is new emphasis on parents' involvement in the running of projects and service. Parents are encouraged to come into the nurseries in the socio-cultural centres, and CAF's work is to help workers accept and encourage this:

> Mme C. at CAF here had worked hard with the . . . workers in their child care training to encourage them to see that parents should come

into and return to the nursery. This is work I continue because . . .
you have to justify what you do, you feel watched and so you often
want them to go. But what I want is to have the reception as far as
possible from the entrance so the parents have to come in and then to
have adult benches for parents to sit down. For four years we've had
difficulties with this in the *halte garderies* I manage and it's true that
it's difficult to have parents sitting there but it's really something
different. [This change] is so that parents remain the educators of their
children, especially in the disadvantaged neighbourhoods, and so that
professionals realise they must work around this.

(Ibid.)

There are problems for school children as well, and rather than let
children simply wander the streets or sit at home in isolation, CAF
provides, and helps associations to provide, activities for them:

There's a lot of reflection in France on the timetable and plan of the
school day. 'Ville' has started a four day week, with no school on
Wednesday. It's becoming a national pattern, but the question becomes
what happens on Wednesdays when the parents work (like many do
on Saturdays). So we need to make children aware of activities and
associations that provide them. . . . The problem may be more children
on the streets and latchkey children.

(Ibid.)

The Centre Communal d'Action Sociale: from assistance to development

'Ville's' Centre Communal d'Action Sociale is within the town hall's
Direction de la Solidarité, with its own social projects and services. The
city's council is committed to promoting local social and economic
development and to do so by maximising partnerships in planning and
by promoting local social ties. Associated with this is the growth in its
own social action by shifting from the old form of stigmatised social
assistance (*aide*) to a system of 'mutualisation'.

The CCAS is an old administrative structure which is completely
maladapted to contemporary changes. At the local level is the person
with needs (families, children, young people, old people, handicapped
people) and the CCAS distributes *aide*. . . . The CCAS social workers
intervene in parallel with those of the social services of the *département* and of CAF . . . they help families who are in difficulty in this

or that expenditure like electricity, food or leisure. . . . But now we try to see that the person isn't 'helped' by being shut in a system that marginalises them by making them dependent on *aide*. That's to say one gives them the means, the power, to do without us, that's our role here.

(M. Naveau, director of CCAS)

The means of achieving this change are partnerships with local associations:

> For the associations which work with us, I'd say they all share the objective that people, whatever their age, take charge of their own problems, so they share the same general philosophy. There are only 6 per cent of elderly people here, so most associations work with young people . . . the organisation of social services is centralised in a certain direction which means they take on at once all ages, families, youth, everyone, so there's a cohesion in policy, because everyone is going in the same direction regarding social development and the principle that inhabitants take part in the decisions taken concerning them, they are actors in the things they do. This is the logic of development rather than assistance.

(Ibid.)

Associations have a particular legal status in France, and the older ones operate like the non-governmental providers of services in Britain. But more recently associations have been a means of promoting and establishing local self-help and residents' groups which can become partners with the city or other agencies in particular spheres. 'Ville' has successfully established the Association pour la Promotion d'Actions de Développement Social.

> It wasn't possible for the city to act on social action and development without a team, so we decided to create an association with some autonomy but with the mission to promote . . . social development, whose logic is to put the inhabitants at the centre and to work with them so that they do things individually and collectively. It's different from the short-term satisfaction of needs where professionals are at the centre. It influences day to day policies. It's connected with other services we run. In my team I have social services, a relatively traditional housing service, a prevention team which works with young people and with the association *Animation Quartier Jeunes* [Neighbourhood Youth Association] and APADES which directly contacts

inhabitants, working on *insertion* and development, making sure that the policies of putting inhabitants at the centre are implemented.

(Ibid.)

APADES is an umbrella association of local groups including a local newspaper, a mobile children's library, a women's group (*La Voix des Femmes*), a theatre group, a credit union, an unemployed group (*Starters*) and it is able, under the direction and funding of the city, to provide opportunities for residents to offer, share or exchange their skills – in redecorating flats, adult literacy and so on and to gain work experience. It operates then as a form of mutual aid, a set of social firms or *services de proximité*, as well as a method of promoting social cohesion of the population. It is directed from the town hall and the CCAS and it employs its own development workers – *agents de développement*. Its work is co-ordinated with that of CAF, for the city funds a high proportion of both, but there is anyway a general climate in which managers expect to be working with colleagues from other agencies and associations and encourage their workers to do so, and workers are attracted to the rich associative life of the city.

The Circonscription d'Action Sociale: balancing child protection and social development

Finally, the *département*'s social services provide a socio-medical service at its Circonscription d'Action Sociale office, where generic social workers or *polyvalentes* (who work in a team with health visitors and midwives) handle most of the statutory work and work more individually with individuals and families with specified difficulties. These are the social workers who have most difficulty in fitting into the new collective approach, for their experience is that they are increasingly submerged in child protection work, and also in the tediously time-consuming work and ever-growing numbers of the contracts with RMI (*Revenu minimum d'insertion*) clients. This is the benefit for the long-term unemployed which requires some kind of commitment to training or loosely conceived work to be agreed to (the *insertion* contract); not surprisingly social workers in the Circonscription d'Action Sociale have the most difficult cases to work with and are becoming increasingly despairing because of the bureaucracy involved. However, APADES associations and the activities at the CAF centre offer opportunities for the *insertion* required in the RMI. Thus we find another point of connection between social workers in a locality, but it is one with pressures on the CAS social workers:

The question that is posed here is the role of the leadership of the municipality in all the actions of development . . . there's a feeling of pressure or constraint among my social work colleagues when asked to participate in this or that action. I would say that this is less true now, the . . . municipality has understood the reality for social workers, there are fewer demands. Up to two years ago APADES had seeemed to think that the non-participation of social work was due to bad will but I think it's changing because the municipality is changing its strategy, so that it wants a good co-ordination of its action with social work. . . . So my colleagues here say *action collective* yes, but don't forget that our priority remains individual work, above all child protection, but also RMI. . . . So for [these] social workers *insertion* means something individual but they use the tools developed by the municipality, for instance the credit union, socio-cultural centres for their users. . . . In the holidays there's *Loisirs Familiaux de Proximité*, in the summer this lets families meet together in the framework of *Pause Café*, another association, and with the support of social workers, they organise the form of holidays, whether daily outings, camping etc., so this creates a good dynamic, and is a tool used by the social workers here for certain families (including those under child protection).

(M. Sauvage, social worker with training as *animateur*, director of CAS)

Social action then operates in a triangle of relationships between the *département* that has the responsibility for social services and which employs qualified social workers for statutory tasks; the commune or city with its social services in the old framework of discretionary assistance, which is once again becoming important but tends not to have qualified social workers or to do statutory work, and CAF or other associations which, by contract, carry out specified statutory or promotional tasks. Social action, then, has shifted from being a field where social workers dominated a passive, scrutinised clientele to one where the the goal is *insertion*, the imaginative search for means of helping people find their own solutions and make their own choices, by working in partnership with other agencies, professionals and associations.

All this has profoundly affected the knowledge base and identity of social work and there is some disagreement as to whether social workers can or should combine statutory child protection responsibilities with social development and collective work (Ion 1993). However, the contemporary intellectual framework behind social action in France would argue that this is not only possible but necessary for society.

SOCIOLOGY AND SOCIAL COHESION: PROMOTING CONVIVIALITY IN THE NEIGHBOURHOOD

As we have seen, although France and the UK have the same labour market problems, fragile and changing family structures, and a concern that Beveridge-style welfare states are failing either to meet or to prevent need, the goals of contemporary policies are different. Those in French social action are overwhelmingly concerned with promoting the well-being of the collectivity while British social welfare concentrates more on the relief of individual need or the control of the dangerous. Yet in both France and England the question of how a society holds together has become more urgent, with unemployment fracturing traditional communities and their cultures, and weakening families.

French social agencies' managers and *élus* are concerned, given their overall mandate of integrated social development, to look at what social workers actually do and how they do it. They tend to use a sociological perspective and this has been strengthened by the fact that many leaders of the social development projects are sociologists, with managers or advisers in social agencies often describing themselves as, by profession, a *sociologue*. Projects (nationally and locally) are evaluated by sociologists (e.g. Estèbe and Donzelot 1993), and advanced training for those in social work and social development is often in university sociology departments.

One sociologist who teaches social workers described the contemporary field as follows:

> When I speak of the destabilised areas, it's not so much the whole territory but certain areas which are in the process of being marginalised. So a solution must be found which concerns persons, social groups and areas, my word for this is development. We need a solution which is positive for persons and also for networks of belonging. While in the 1960s *le social* was the business of social work, today we need a mobilisation of social work with *élus* and business leaders. Everyone . . . is aware that there's a problem to resolve. What I note is that today the frontiers and limits are blurring between the status and role of professionals and other social actors . . .

> The term 'bottom-up development' is used as a contrast to 'top down development' from the state. At the end of the twentieth century what interests me is the combination of both movements, for instance in urban development in neighbourhoods, this doesn't simply come from above, the associative movements and municipal policies are very interesting and reciprocally the policies of the state are put into

practice at local level. So I don't think in France there's the obsession with the sharing of power with people (as in empowerment strategies), rather we are looking for an articulation between a relevant social policy and a bottom-up movement. Personally I believe we need this, we need both ... so there has to be an articulation between the state, local collectivities, associations, professions, which support local people, networks of partnership, associations.

> (M. Troussier, sociologist who teaches in a social work college)

In describing how he manages his social workers in this time of change, M. Cardi said

> I use my training as a sociologist and I try to help professionals understand this new landscape and the changes in their classical function and to understand how their professional practice has to change to be effective in this new landscape. So it's a kind of technical support. . . . The working week of 40 hours is disappearing. People hope or believe that work will reappear and people are helped to find work and believe in it. In other words, we have to think of social intervention in relation to the evolution of the whole of society. . . . Strategies of *socialisation* must find new mechanisms. That's extremely complicated and it's what I try to do, it's almost a work of research, very long and difficult with no landmarks, no theory of its own, all has to be found, and I've tried to find how *socialisation* functioned around social exchange. . . . The hypothesis is that social exchange can't replace work but it can help people.
>
> (M. Cardi, sociologist and manager in a family welfare agency)

His agency both develops and provides services of *animation* and uses them in helping a range of social workers and other professionals adapt their skills and thinking. Social work, he says, has to move from being a crutch (as it was in the *assistance* mode) to being a form of social advice, and *animateurs* move from being providers of activities in a structured setting to

> something much more open and experimental; what is common is that the people themselves take charge of their affairs and try to negotiate in their own way – which is local social development or *animation locale*.
>
> (Ibid.)

He sees sociology as providing the concepts needed to underpin this work. A sociological perspective of the 1990s is being put into practice:

we are not only invited to consider demographic factors, the social impact of the changes in labour markets, and so forth, but cultural factors. Modern social thought is stressing the possibility that, without stable employment, the working class – the backbone of French solidarity – will lose its coherence based on work cultures and communities. Furthermore, a society thus enfeebled is threatened by American TV and films. The Frenchman or woman or child's senses of belonging and identity are simultaneously weakened and corrupted, so that anomie and isolation are fertile ground for the negative messages of American media culture – individualism, short-termism, greed, violence:

> Everyone says the people, the users must be actors, but few do anything about it. Two reasons: (1) political reasons – power – some gain power from representing the people (including social workers); (2) 'poor people' in their variety: their lives are lived through TV images. This prevents thought because people think only through images which they have in the front of their heads as to what they should do. It's striking that people live TV and American series and project themselves into Dallas etc. . . . All the work done is not just to help them, not just to rediscover their own roots, but little by little to reconstitute their social personality. . . . In other words the perspective of social work is to recreate social identities in people, and it's very fragile these days.
>
> (Ibid.)

This view, in official discourse and in social practice, of the crisis as an economic crisis and as a cultural crisis shapes much of what social workers actually do. Youth centres and centres for families and children are centred on the professional field of the socio-cultural. We still find traditional social work in these centres – counselling and psychotherapeutic work with individuals or families with specific and serious difficulties. But the broader setting is one which seeks to attract local people into centres for a range of shared leisure activities, which works with local groups to develop neighbourhood social ties. At the same time the centres offer their users tangible outcomes such as holidays and outings together, and develop forms of supported mutual aid. Leisure and cultural activities then are seen as more than just the prevention of delinquency or family problems, as is often the case in the UK. They are seen as important to the development of social ties and the promotion of cultural identities and senses of belonging, which, while recognising the identities of ethnic minorities, also centre on the idea of being French – and of belonging to particular regions of the European Union.

The notion of conviviality then is important in French social practice. Asked who and what *animation* is for, Mme Feret, director of the 'Ville' *centre socio-culturel*, said:

Above all, for families, but also for children and young people. We work with 'Ville' and with the schools ... the *animateurs* who work with adults concentrate on leisure, for instance going on holiday – the *loisirs de proximité* and *vacances familles*, as well as do-it-yourself for decorating and repairing things in the home. There is also the catering in the centre, for some conviviality when groups decide to stay and eat together after their groups. We concentrate on the home as well as in the larger sense on *l'habitat*, on living in the neighbourhood and the city.

(Mme Feret, social worker and director of *centre socio-culturel*)

The social workers in the centre are encouraged to do the same, to get to know their families in a different way from that in their child protection role, and to provide their clients with a different kind of action:

The work here includes outings like climbing and we have worked with women who are very strong yet who had not imagined themselves doing such things and we showed them photos of themselves to change their self-images. We also went to the sea, with women who had never worn bathing costumes because they thought they were too fat, etc., so that also let us work with people on the qualities of their personal life, their body, their city, their diet; through our catering service, people share their lives, discuss a lot and make ties.

(Ibid.)

This strong French emphasis on conviviality and social cohesion explains the place of the *services de proximité* in French social policy. These 'social firms' (to use an English term), a sector mid-way between public and private, are sometimes referred to in France as *l'économie solidaire*. These organisations are not just a new way of meeting today's new needs and demands – notably for early child care and for care for elderly people (but also care of the environment, leisure, arts, culture and so forth). Nor are they just a means of creating 'work' (whether paid, voluntary, as work experience, as training or as service while on benefit). They are a means of promoting social cohesion because they tie services more closely to the world and needs of users (they are above all local); they create new partnerships between social movements, associations, voluntary organisations and the local state; and they thus promote the healthy development of that sphere between state and market, and between public and private – civil society (Laville 1992: 18–23).

This view of the significance of *services de proximité* underpins, as we have seen, Ville's network of associations and CAF's work with neighbourhood groups. It is the reason for CAF moving closer to the parents' movement in early child care, supporting the *crèches parentales*. These grew from the 1968 student movement (like their German counterparts – see Gerzer-Sass and Pettinger, Chapter 6 in this book, and see Laville 1992: 29–33). This movement wanted more than to fill the gaps in public child care; it sought to develop collective settings for children's socialisation which retained parental responsibility and involvement. While it created links and networks between parents in neighbourhoods, it was also looking for a new pedagogy – a blend of care and education which moved away from the old hierarchical, formal, rigid routines in the nurseries of not so long ago. It meant responding more individually to children's needs, and seeing learning and development as growing from everyday life activities rather than from strict medical or 'educational' practices. The original *crèches sauvages* (unofficial crèches) of the parents' movement have recently strongly influenced formal providers such as CAF, which have been reminded by the growth of the parents' movement at both national and local levels of the need to work with parents. CAF now agrees that it is as much the professional child care workers as the parents who need training, which helps them to work in partnership and to provide flexible child care services. At the same time they are capitalising on the movement in the drive to build local social cohesion.

Social action in contemporary France then is concerned above all with social integration and with working collectively with groups of local people, children, youth and adults, to promote that integration. It valorises and encourages group activities – holidays, outings, eating together – which centre on participation in the public sphere. It seeks to develop the neighbourhood as the new locus of solidarity now that the workplace cannot be so.

What of participation by users and residents? Clearly a central principle in social development, this is the area which is most problematic in the French schemes, whose success story lies rather in strategic planning at national and at local levels, and in the partnerships of professionals with associations at local levels. There is much rhetoric about involving users but descriptions of how projects actually run and of local planning show that residents and users tend to be outnumbered by a multiplicity of experts. So while the success of the French schemes is sometimes described as its combining of top-down and bottom-up development, the bottom-up side of the equation is less democratic than the rhetoric suggests, indeed it has been described as a new Jacobinism given the powerful new caste of mayors and *élus* it has empowered. There are employment opportunities for those, including social workers who can speak for residents, users, inhabitants, and a degree of competition to be the ones to be heard and to take legitimacy from this. On the other hand social workers have often stood apart from the big social development and *insertion* schemes, saying that, for all the rhetoric of being centred on the user and the local inhabitant, it remains the experts who prescribe what the good society should look like and how to get there.

CONCLUSION: SOCIAL DEVELOPMENT – A NEW PARADIGM?

My general view is that, despite some serious problems, the French attempt to promote the social welfare of (and with) children, youth and families in the context of social development is one we must learn from. Social development is viewed in France as the paradigm for a future welfare state, tackling as it does the connected issues of citizenship, employment, exclusion, the quality of neighbourhood life and the changing structures and ties of family.

In contrast to the curbs on the powers of local government over the last fifteen years in Britain, we see a more powerful local and regional system of government emerging in France which can begin to offer some of the hopes of 'thinking global, acting local'. Importantly too it is expanding the number of people with a stake in good provision of local services, with a say in the form of those services, and with the ability and power to negotiate and contract with the national state for resources. For all the branches of social work in France, however, the task, as they know it and understand it, is to expand this notion of democracy by continuously working to find ways of involving users and residents, and to ensure that they have a say in the nature of the good society. While social workers in the statutory social services departments need to ensure that they are not being set up to fail, with too much being expected of them, the independent sector and the cities' communes are showing how family support and social development can be combined.

The French schemes are a huge experiment in getting agencies and professionals to integrate the principles of social development into their work. The central concept of *insertion* introduces a way of working that points to the environment rather than the person as the source of problems. Work with children and families focuses on their environment, because their citizenship is understood as existing in or being threatened in the public sphere. Helping people to participate in political, social and cultural ways in their localities is a goal in its own right – to prevent the fracturing of society, but also as the best means of supporting the private sphere of the family. For too long social work in the UK has focused on the private sphere and its pathologies; social policy and social work need to learn from France and move into the more public sphere if it is genuinely to promote and support children, young people and their families.

REFERENCES

Cannan, C. (1995) 'Urban social development in France', *Community Development Journal*, 30, 3: 238–47.
CNAF (Caisse Nationale des Allocations Familiales) (1992) *Les Orientations de l'Action Sociale Familiale des CAF 1992-1996*, Paris: CNAF.
Corbillon, M. (1993) 'France', in M. J. Colton and W. Hellinckx (eds), *Child Care in the E.C.: A Country-Specific Guide to Foster and Residential Care*, Aldershot: Arena/Aldgate Publishing.
Estèbe, P. and Donzelot, J. (1993) 'Le développement social urbain: est-il une politique? Les leçons de l'évaluation', *Regards sur l'Actualité*, 196: 29–38.
Ion, J (1993) 'Les métiers du social à l'épreuve de l'exclusion', *Regards sur l'Actualité*, 196: 39–49.
Laville, J.-L (1992) *Les Services de Proximité en Europe*, Paris: Syros Alternatives.
Le Galès, P. and Mawson, P. (1994) *Management Innovations in Urban Policy – Lessons From France*, Luton: Local Government Management Board.
Silver, H. (1994) *Social Exclusion and Social Solidarity: Three Paradigms*, Geneva: International Institute for Labour Studies.

Chapter 5

Family support and the journey to empowerment

Chris Warren

Family support practice means promoting social support networks for children and their families within a range of formal and informal organisations. There is a growing acknowledgement that lack of social support networks increases risk (Camasso and Camasso 1986), and that the promotion of social supports enhances opportunity for citizenship, which is to say opportunities to participate reasonably, to play accepted social roles and to take responsibility (Cochran 1985; Kagan *et al.* 1987). An evaluation of family support practice in the voluntary child welfare sector (DoH 1992–5) has identified a practice which resembles empowerment practice. In this chapter I attempt a focused account of empowerment practice in which I want to emphasise what I call the empowerment journey, and I report on a small study that brings to life some challenges for practitioners. I shall start with two examples of the empowerment journey, one personal (a fictional account constructed from experiences of young people), the other structural.

1   Ann, age 14, is the main carer in her family, caring for the physical needs of her disabled mother and playing a major role in the day to day care of her three younger siblings. Her school attendance is very erratic. She heard about the Young Carers' Project through the school network. She bravely called into the project office one day, and liked and developed a trusting relationship with a project worker. Much later, the pleasure of involvement in a recreational summer group led her to join a regular group of other young carers. Over time, cautiously, she and her family became less resistant to sharing with other agencies attention to the needs of her mother and siblings. Ann participated in project development meetings and, once, spoke at a young carers' conference. Two years on, Ann was an altogether more confident person, with some wider friendships, and some educational opportunities gained. The

project had engaged Ann well, cared for her, encouraged her socially and had helped her to participate and represent herself.

2   The Oakshire project constructs its intervention from a number of perspectives; the needs of the child, the parent and child relationship, the parent's own personal development and the parent as participant in community affairs. There are three workers. The outreach worker, receiving her referrals mainly from health visitors, focuses on the relationship needs of parent and child. The group worker concentrates on the support of women in different groups, as well as the pre-school experience of their children. And the community worker enables parents in partnership with child care professionals to organise to press for universal child care facilities in their area. What seems important here is not that each parent has direct experience of each aspect of the project – they generally do not – but it is the positive impact of the structure on the project workers whose particular focus has equal status within the project, and the fact that the needs of parents and children are represented in the structure of the project.

THE CHILDREN ACT 1989 AND FAMILY SUPPORT

A series of British research studies in the 1980s (DHSS 1985) encouraged a critique of social work practice to the effect that child rescue had become the dominant principle of child care social work. That is to say, practice was beginning to turn its back on the child's original family. It had become, so the argument went, overdependent upon legal frameworks rather than negotiation, and insufficiently sensitive to the competing needs of family members. Thus one major intention of the legislation was to encourage negotiation between social worker and client. The 1989 Act gave a broad definition of a 'child in need' and made it a duty for local authorities to provide a range of services to protect and to safeguard the welfare of such children. Another device – Section 1(5) – which discourages intervention based on judicial means, unless absolutely necessary – presses social workers to derive their mandate from negotiation. The debate has continued, transforming itself into the 1990s. How can we slow down the child protection juggernaut? We do not want to discard the best of our knowledge and practice in protecting children, it is generally argued, but we want change such that social work with children and their families can represent itself and be identified in the minds of the public with broader activities, for example, family support.

Part 3 and Schedule 2 of the Children Act 1989 provides for a range of family support services. This is elaborated in Guidance to the Act and its origin is described by Rose in Gibbons (1992).

Section 17 (10) of the Children Act 1989 reads,

For the purposes of this part a child shall be taken to be in need if

(a) he is unlikely to achieve or maintain, or to have the opportunity of achieving or maintaining, a reasonable standard of health or development without the provision for him of services by a local authority under this Part;

(b) his health or development is likely to be significantly impaired, or further impaired, without the provision for him of such services; or

(c) he is disabled.

This is a definition provided by the Act and the local authority is expected to provide a range of services for children in need in their area, to consult widely about their provision, and to monitor. The local authority should, in the words of the Act: 'safeguard and promote the welfare of children within their area who are in need'.

Such a range of family support services is specifically aimed at keeping children within their families. Moreover, this legislation allows for services to be provided for other family members and people significant to the child if the child in need will benefit. The 'targets' of such services are therefore many and varied. This is a major difference from previous legislation. The local authority can protect children from current or future harm either by providing family support services under Part 3 of the Act or, if the additional criteria based on harm are met, by satisfying the court that a compulsory order is necessary. Thus family support is linked to protection.

Practice outcomes of the legislation

Within this legal umbrella two practices – partnership practice and family support practice – which offer broader frameworks in which to locate practice have become the focus of attention.

Partnership practice, it has been argued, underpins all aspects of the Children Act (FRG 1991; Marsh and Fisher 1992). Partnership is not solely a word of welfare, and has been favoured particularly by government since 1979. Within welfare, Marsh and Fisher have set down the principles of partnership as follows:

investigation of problems must be with the explicit consent of the potential user(s) and client(s);

user agreement or a clear statutory mandate are the only bases of
partnership-based intervention;
intervention must be based upon the views of all relevant family members
and carers;
services must be based on negotiated agreement, rather than on assumptions and/or prejudices concerning the behaviour and wishes of users;
users must have the greatest possible degrees of choice in the services
that they are offered.

(Marsh and Fisher 1992: 13–14)

These principles are then developed in terms of direct practice skills, with
an emphasis on active participation, task-centred, joint record-keeping,
clear mandate and full information.

Family support practice was given early expression in Britain by, for
example, Goldberg and Sinclair (1986), sharing many aspects of an
already established movement in North America. They ordered their ideas
in terms of individual, group, day care and multiple approaches. They
identified befriending practices, self-help initiatives such as Scope, Opus,
Cope and family centres which they considered under their heading of
multiple approaches. Gibbons (1992) looks ahead and reviews ideas about
family support that have emerged from the debate about the Children Act
1989, and which have become enshrined in Part 3, Schedule 2 of the Act.
Most authors find the concept of *prevention* wanting and seek better things
from its re-formulation – *promotion* – in family support (Rose 1992).

In the USA, Kagan *et al.* (1987) provide accounts of the development
of what might genuinely be called a family support movement in the USA,
and which appears to have lessons for the UK. Various authors look back
to and beyond the US's own 'Children Act' (PL 1980–292) in their
review, and most authors point to roots in the settlement movement
(community work), early education programmes like Head Start, and
self-help action.

THE FAMILY SUPPORT INITIATIVE

In my evaluation of seven family support projects, as part of the
Department of Health Family Support Initiative (DoH 1992–5), one task
was to understand the boundary of family support. What is this range of
services? Is it possible to talk meaningfully about family support
practice? To what extent do the ideas behind family support compare and
contrast with ideas about prevention and empowerment? How do you
categorise family support services?

It was decided to use a framework of family support developed by Carl Dunst (1990) whose review of American family support literature enabled him to propose an evaluation framework which may be applied both to policy and to practice. By applying Dunst to our seven family support projects we sought to gain some understanding of its use as well as raise or confirm evaluation questions to be tackled.

Dunst identified six major sets of family support principles:

1 Enhancing a sense of community.
2 Mobilising resources and supports.
3 Shared responsibility and collaboration.
4 Protecting family integrity.
5 Strengthening family functioning.
6 Proactive human service practices.

The family support scale was completed by practitioners in all seven of the projects we evaluated. Dunst's family support principles extended our view of practice beyond those of partnership and, explicitly and implicitly, connected with the culture of practice amongst the seven projects of our evaluation. However, the word which practitioners are likely to employ as much as, if not rather more than, either partnership or family support practice is *empowerment*.

Empowerment practice

The word 'empowerment' appears to be part of the common discourse of social work students, local practitioners and managers, and the population of practitioners who have participated as respondents in our project evaluations. The word 'empowerment' for them seems to sum up the aspiration of social and community work. However, the word empowerment does appear to be used indiscriminately. In a lively bulletin dedicated to debate about empowerment practice in family support, Rappoport, whilst suggesting barriers to the development of empowerment practice – he cites individualism, professional socialisation, racism, sexism and the functions of both state and non-governmental organisations – also cautions that 'Given our power to legitimate, we need to be more critical and less casual about what we advocate as empowering' (Rappoport 1995).

I propose that whilst partnership practice is the bedrock of 'good practice', and supports empowerment practice, it is not the same as empowerment. Empowerment is a rather more distinctive activity which has its roots in a radical feminist perspective, a combination of the humanist counselling perspective on the one hand and a collective process of politicisation on the other (Howe 1987).

The empowerment literature

There is a substantial US literature on empowerment practice. Such practice has its parallels in Europe in the tradition of cultural animation (Reisch *et al.* 1981). In the UK there is a growing literature on empowerment which makes a solid claim to be part of the social work (Parsloe and Stevenson 1993) and community work agendas (Craig *et al.* 1990). In UK social work – where two increasingly separate cultures of service delivery are being constructed, one for children and families and one for 'adults' – the term empowerment has been applied particularly to services at the social work/health interface concerning the needs of adults – elders, those with learning disabilities, physical disabilities and mental ill-health (Barker and Peck 1987; Brechan *et al.* 1981; Holdsworth 1991; see chapter by Peter Durrant in this book). One exception is the increasing interest in the UK in the New Zealand Whanau Family Group Method (Connolly 1989, see chapter by Jo Tunnard in this book). In US literature there has been a greater connection of empowerment practice to supporting children and their families.

Three perspectives of empowerment practice summarised

The first perspective (Berger and Neuhaus 1977)) highlights the part played by mediating structures in communities both as venues for participation and as vehicles for projecting a set of values. The implication is a practice that is organisationally and inter-organisationally focused. Such a practice will prioritise those organisations that most reflect traditional values.

The second perspective (Dunst *et al.* 1994) is more developed and establishes a set of principles and premises that share common ground with a range of empowerment theorists, not least the assumption of an ecological perspective (Bronfenbrenner 1979) as a paradigm for understanding human behaviour. Dunst and associates provide a unitary framework, an analytical tool which helps to set a manageable agenda for further study.

The third perspective enhances others by its emphasis on process, making the links between levels of work and collective methods. This perspective has never really departed from the framework developed by Solomon (1987) and many other theorists (Guttierrez 1990; Reisch *et al.*

1981; Barber 1991; Parsons 1991; Mullender and Ward 1991; Freeman *et al.* 1992). Briefly, oppression which is experienced over time becomes internalised and the individual is prevented from carrying out the ordinary participative tasks of citizenship; for example, work, education, being a parent. Solomon calls them indirect blocks. Direct blocks are also experienced; for example, poor services, poor and unhealthy neighbourhoods, discrimination. Thus to recover my position as a disempowered person I need (a) to know what has been done to me and (b) to embark on a journey both to externalise the problem as well as to take responsibility for my own 'recovery'.

It is particularly the emphasis on process and collective practice which marks out this third perspective. It is argued that only through collective involvement am I likely to identify support over time and to discover and externalise my plight. Individual support, whether through therapy, counselling or advocacy, is not precluded but is identified as an element in the journey. Thus such an approach is best implemented within broad programmes rather than by individual and small-scale initiatives. Moreover, it is argued that individuals gain their empowerment; it is not a gift, so to speak, handed out by professionals. They can only aid and abet in the process; their job is, rather, to facilitate, set a climate (Simon 1990). How then do you construct such a climate? I will elaborate Dunst's framework and then build on important emphases by Cochran, particularly the idea of empowerment as process (Cochran 1985).

Dunst *et al.* (1994) offer a matrix with which to analyse empowerment. A review of empowerment literature leads Dunst and colleagues to enumerate six ways in which empowerment has been given meaning.

1 *Empowerment as philosophy.* The authors draw on Rappoport's three guiding principles of an empowerment philosophy, which are:

- all people have existing strengths and capabilities as well as the capacity to become more competent;
- the failure of a person to display competence is *not* due to deficits within a person but rather the failure of social systems to provide or create opportunities for competencies to be displayed or acquired; and,
- in situations where existing capabilities need to be strengthened or new competencies need to be learned, they are best learned through experiences that lead people to make self-attributions about their capabilities to influence important life events.

2 *Empowerment as a paradigm.* Here a distinction is drawn between treatment, prevention and promotion models. Promotion models draw on a particular language – e.g. mastery, optimisation, competencies and

capabilities, proactive, strength-based. In contrast, the language of both treatment and prevention models is said to be deficit- or problem-based – e.g. poor functioning, poor parenting, preventing poor parenting, preventing family breakdown.

3   *Empowerment as process.* Here the focus is upon empowering experiences over time which acknowledge that confidence and competence are not gained quickly. Moreover, it embraces key elements in a journey, engagement, mentoring, reflective action, resources, collective support, etc.

4   *Empowerment as partnership.* Here empowerment is seen as an inter-personal construct, relational power sharing. The important dimension of empowerment as partnership is in the experience of the individual of a particular transaction. The emphasis on the experience, the history created of something good coming out of a relationship which was *felt* to be collaborative is important.

5   *Empowerment as performance.* Here the focus is on what has been learnt. What do you need to be able to do to build resource networks, for example?

6   *Empowerment as perception.* This is a focus on the cognitive dimension and connects with measures which variously travel under the heading of self-esteem.

Dunst and associates provide a unitary tool to consider empowerment practice, adding two other dimensions: context, based on Bronfenbrenner's (1979) eco-systemic model; and four levels – individual, group, organisation and community (Dunst *et al.* 1994: 23).

The third perspective, represented by the Cornell Empowerment Group (Cochran 1985, 1987; Cochran and Brassard 1979; Cochran and Henderson 1990), helps us to think about making the links between levels. It emphasises three cornerstones of empowerment practice: process; mutual respect; critical reflection.

Process

This perspective, whilst acknowledging that empowerment can be thought of in terms of both outcome and process, lays special emphasis on process. It is argued that outcomes can be seen as stepping stones in the process. I find it helpful to talk of a journey. Theorists cite the work of Keiffer (1984) who sees empowerment as a long-term and continuing process of adult development. Keiffer proposes four stages in an individual's empowerment story, which are described as 'era of entry';

'era of advancement'; 'era of incorporation', and the 'era of commit-ment'. Moreover, Keiffer's findings tell us that individuals' journeys through these 'eras' can take a minimum of four years (a theme we are at pains to emphasise in this book). Moreover, according to Keiffer, an important outcome of empowerment is effective citizenship.

Mutual respect

The second broad cornerstone of this perspective is mutual respect, a principle shared by most commentators. But here it is developed as follows, including:

1 A focus on power – a desire to share it and devolve it, as well as to understand its transactional character. Thus we come to see power played out at myriad levels, e.g. resources, gender, economic oppor-tunity, within families, communities, etc. (Pinderhughes 1983; Hasen-field 1987).
2 An acknowledgement of the adaptive capacity of people and thus the need to identify and develop their strengths (already well developed for example by Maluccio et al. 1986).
3 An emphasis on diversity, history and culture. This follows from the ecological perspective. It connects well also with anti-discriminatory practice.
4 Users/clients must play the primary role. This is a principle generally shared but fiendishly difficult to honour.
5 Programmes should be located at local and community level.

Critical reflection

Here we see a re-emergence of Freire's work in, for example, French, US and British literature (Freynet 1995; Reisch et al. 1981; Mullender and Ward 1991) in which, through collectivity and discourse, people are enabled to distance themselves from their predicament in order to come to an understanding of the way they are prevented from citizenship. This is an approach based in ideas of adult education and cultural animation, more at home in a European than in an Anglo-Saxon tradition.

Related to this perspective is an emphasis on (a) rights, the acknowl-edgement of a lack of resources at society level (b) an enabling political framework – intervention is more effective when permission is given through policies, funding and an enabling political climate; (c) and caring. As well as the importance of peer group support, theorists underline the need for a 'mentor', a confidential one-to-one relationship, particularly at the beginning of the journey.

A STUDY OF EMPOWERMENT PRACTICE

I constructed a semi-structured questionnaire based on this perspective (see Appendix) and invited practitioners from five of the projects participating in our Family Support Initiative Evaluation to reflect on their 'empowerment' practice. The participating projects were all located in national voluntary organisations.

The Oakshire Project (parent and child) was based in a small town that had been devastated by structural unemployment. Three workers – outreach worker, group worker and community worker – sought to integrate practices of counselling, group work and community development on behalf of parents and children. (This was similar to the original model of Solomon's project, through which she developed her empowerment theory.) The outreach worker visited families in their homes, designing programmes with parents (mostly women) to overcome issues in early childhood – sleeplessness, control, toilet training, aggression and so on, The group worker ran various support groups for parents, and parents and children. And the community worker, who was also the project manager, initiated and facilitated a community group in its quest for a parent and child centre.

The Hornbeam Project (family health) took place in a large, multi-ethnic, inner-city estate. Here a worker and a number of sessional workers, in alliance with other workers, for example the race equality unit, sought to identify families with children and young people who had disabilities or chronic ill-health and develop opportunities individually and collectively for them. Significant outcomes included a number of self-help groups based on health themes; for example, depression, anxiety and asthma. Community research was a distinctive feature of the project, representing the health needs of families through the local democratic process.

The Hazel Project operated across several local authority areas. Here the organisation experimented with the provision of a foster carer as refuge and carer for mother and child, victims of male violence. The project complemented the work of local refuges by offering care to mothers with small children and to users referred from a local street drugs project. The work involved reframing as a family-violence approach what might hitherto have been seen as a child protection matter. The focus was particularly on parent and child and their nurture, at the beginning of the break from a violent male partner. Future outcomes would involve recruiting more family carers as a collective of support for themselves and potentially the families who used them.

To encourage different parent groups, the Yew Project developed a trigger video to encourage different parent groups based on issues emerging from the early years. Using the organisation's extensive national network of toy libraries, day care centres and parents' projects, the trainer (reporting to an alliance of parents and professionals) embarked on developing groups amongst parents. Whilst much early energy was concerned with the video, its later application drew the project into collective practices with parents using centres as springboards for action.

The Northshire Project engaged young carers, offered individual support and opportunities, and endeavoured to influence service systems that could help them. This project reflected a children's rights perspective (see Clifton and Hodgson's chapter in this book). Three project workers worked alongside young people whose family role was as carer, often the lynchpin in a family where parent or parents suffered major ill-health and disability. Young carers suffer conflicts in their responsibility to their families and their personal and educational needs as young people in their own right. Activities meant involvement of young people in the heart of the project, including policy and staff recruitment. It involved personal support for young people, young carers' groups, disseminating research undertaken about the needs of such young people, encouraging similar project development in the region, and enabling young carers to speak out, for example at conferences. The project also sought a sensitive response from local authorities whose mandate for such young people included a potentially problematic cross-over of two major pieces of legislation, the NHS and Community Care Act 1990 and the Children Act 1989.

The responses of project workers

Practitioners had no difficulty in reflecting on power imbalance or ideas of internalised oppression. They identified men's power in families and they consistently saw the process of self-blame amongst women as a particular feature of their work. In meeting together, young people encountered differences in expectations about their role according to different ethnic and other cultures. For young people, knowing you have missed out, wanting an education, being a young woman in a male environment were stressed. Identifying and exploiting community resources highlighted insufficiency of resources, and networking was put forward as a basic skill to be used in this domain.

Partnership practice on the basis of shared decision making with users was well articulated and assimilated (there were many examples of written agreements) though strengths-based practice was less well expressed. Keeping users in the driving seat elicited enthusiastic agreement, though two highlighted conflicts where there was a compulsory mandate – a court order – and also there were dilemmas for group workers managing over-dominant members.

Critical reflection – the emphasis on peer groups as the primary means of helping people to understand the external origins to problems and to act on this knowledge – is regarded as desirable by respondents but is not seen as a *sine qua non* of practice. Most practitioners do have a goal of helping users to participate in groups though much experience is in working with and supporting individuals. Examples given remind us that the process of individual support, through to group participation, through to community participation, is not straightforward or indeed linear in the way outlined. The empowerment journey as identified by the experiences of these projects is a long and uneven one.

Practitioners underlined the strength of enabling users to opt in and out of the programme at various stages. There were some gratifying examples of users moving on into work and education. Young people in particular saw education as a route to liberty. Some practitioners expressed the problem of managing dependency whether individually or in the group. Caring for people drew constructive comment about the role of support groups (and, in passing, the problems of managing the anger of users about their treatment from established agencies). Practitioners expressed some confusion as to whether they should adopt the mentor role or whether and how they should encourage users to gain this help from the wider community. Responses were unfocused here although in all five projects the role of individual support of users as part of the beginning of the empowerment journey was a substantial part of practice.

Responses to questions about rights and responsibilities varied in their precision. Interestingly, it elicited reflections on the rights and responsibilities of parenthood, the re-ordering of roles in families – for example, in ill-health – and the dilemmas for practitioners in being cast in parent roles by users. Citizenship – the rights and opportunities which enable people to break away from being stuck on the margins of society – is not generally part of the discourse of practitioners. They do not automatically talk about citizenship as a goal of practice, except established community workers who are more versed in such language and debate. One identified denial of the disabled living allowance as a denial of citizenship.

Bronfenbrenner's latter-day emphasis on the need for challenge coupled with support drew varying understanding. Practitioners used the word challenge differently, in managing authority, as a tactic in anti-discriminatory practice, and as opportunity. Mutual respect was strongly expressed and articulated. Responses included the need for and useful-ness of written policies in organisations, struggling with users' hostilities towards some agencies, working with different religious beliefs and cultural practices, the time needed to establish a code of ethics in group work, and the need for realism in expectations. Listening to young people, engaging them in staff recruitment, for example, has had a profoundly important effect on the Young Carers' Project.

CONCLUSION

In this chapter I have outlined some perspectives of empowerment practice and reflected on the practices of those working in some voluntary-sector family support projects. In this chapter a focused empowerment theory proposes that intervention must make available a number of key opportunities and form the components of an empowerment journey: engagement, individual support, support/care from peer group, critical reflection within a peer group, taking action, citizenship through par-ticipation.

Overall, practitioners use the word empowerment extensively and through their practice demonstrate an intuitive attachment to aspects reflected in the literature. Areas which are particularly strong are those described as values and assumptions. (This is well developed in Hulyer's chapter in this book.) Values are the starting point. However, identifying the stages of an empowerment journey is more problematic. Unlike Keiffer, I was not able to track the particular journeys of individuals. And, for the most part, practitioners expressed a commitment to em-powerment in individual work. Constructing an intervention based on all stages of the empowerment journey has a number of challenging implications.

First, it involves a complicated structure. Some family centres seem to manage it, though one or other end of the continuum seems to dominate, managing risk on the one hand, encouraging participation on the other. Whether the key elements of empowerment are built into one project, or between several projects (programme), or as part of what might be called a configuration of services in the community, a central challenge is to make the links between them.

Another issue concerns practitioner roles, and matters of needs, rights and expertise. Some of the practitioners in the study have reflected on their attempts at achieving equality in their worker–user relationship. The literature of disability in particular talks of handing over power and expertise, in an equal relationship. Here the assumptions are that users define their needs entirely and the practitioner has the technical task to hand over the goods. Is this all there is to it? What of valuing and using expertise? Moreover, in each stage of the empowerment process there are dimensions of inequality. For example, the power you have as counsellor or mentor, the power vested in the facilitator in the group-joining phase, the powerful knowledge of the experienced networker, the power of the educator and so on. It seems to me that what is important turns on how such power is negotiated. We expect such responsibility and discretion from professionals, and this is an important focus of professional education.

In similar vein, one respondent saw managing compulsory orders and child protection procedures as a challenge to empowerment practice. It does not have to be. Note how Marsh and colleagues have sought to define partnership practice within a compulsory mandate (Marsh and Fisher 1992). What is also important is that (a) practitioners acknowledge they have only a part to play in the journey; (b) practitioners assume responsibility for sign-posting so that users can take advantage of other parts of the system; (c) programmes themselves need to provide varieties of opportunity.

Another issue concerns the journey from support to action and the traditions and capacities of practitioners. As an example, I refer to the potentially different group-work agendas of social workers and community workers. The primary agenda of the social work group might arguably be seen as an expressive one. That is to say, it is primarily concerned with members' emotional support and the group's capacity to nurture and strengthen members. On the other hand, the primary agenda of the community work group may be described as an instrumental one. That is to say the group's main concerns are external and matters of nurture and support are only important insofar as they serve the external goals of the group. Valued roles in such groups will include leadership, and a range of technical skills and knowledge related to the external needs of the group. It can mean two different activities facilitated by practitioners from very different traditions. This may have polarised the position somewhat but I do believe it demonstrates the considerable polarity between social work and community work perspectives, which is consistently underestimated.

What the empowerment journey proposes is to bring together both these perspectives; it combines the care and counselling perspective with the collective and the political (as expressed for example in Freire (1972)). It is akin to what Howe calls the radical humanist perspective, signalled at the start of this chapter. There are many implications. Can the same practitioner embrace this continuum of practice? Does it need different practitioners and if so, who pulls it together and keeps it in balance? Does current training encourage this blend of skills? It involves reviewing training in social and community work and, in particular, a rejection of the narrow world of current practice-learning opportunities in social work. I believe it should involve constructing curricula based on the empowerment structure, emphasising group practice, working in transitions, working in community-based initiatives, and linking welfare concerns with universal needs. In the domain of children and families this means ensuring a range of experience for trainees, from direct work with children, to parent and child work, to addressing a variety of parent needs (personal and emotional, educational, as active participants and so on). It also involves broad-based partnership training initiatives across localities and neighbourhoods.

In my still elementary attempts at testing this empowerment model my attention is consistently drawn to the word synergy. I met it – *synergie* – often in the original French text on which Chapter 10, 'Think global, act local', is based. The dictionary has it as: the combined effect of drugs, organs, etc., that exceeds the sum of their individual effects. (From the Greek *sunergos*, working together.) So often family centre workers will describe to me how their combination of the practical and the therapeutic, day care, education and information, networking, sign-posting and community outreach – in many ways an empowerment structure – develops an impetus, a sense of confidence and effectiveness which cannot be explained by the individual components of the centre. My guess is that practitioners who combine to work in this way are strong team members, good at transitions and making the links, and are able to look beyond the focus of their own specific practice. It would be good to know more about these matters as part of a more hopeful, though no less complicated, future agenda for children and families social action.

APPENDIX: EMPOWERMENT QUESTIONNAIRE

Empowerment questionnaire – a checklist for practitioners, students and practice teachers

Use this to evaluate your intervention with a particular client or group. Best done several times, and even better at the beginning and end of a particular intervention. Also best done with co-worker, supervisor, evaluator. Suggest scoring where 1 = a long way to go and 7 = excellent. Scoring is not valid as a comparison between people but can be usefully employed as an opener and as a measure over time. Ask yourself each question in respect of your client/family/group, and use the right-hand column to do a quick score and note an example.

1 Power   1–2–3–4–5–6–7
Can begin to understand and discuss the nature
of power imbalance at both a psychological (e.g.
the family background, gender, age) and at the
structural level (e.g. denied access to decent
housing, environment, work).
(Hasenfield 1987; Pinderhughes 1983)

2 Internalisation of oppression   1–2–3–4–5–6–7
Can begin to understand and discuss the way in
which past oppression can be internalised,
resulting in poor self-image, de-skilling, etc.
(Solomon 1987)

3 Identifying resources   1–2–3–4–5–6–7
View the community as an oasis of potential
resources for consumers rather than as an
obstacle.
(Parsloe and Stevenson 1993)

4 Strengths   1–2–3–4–5–6–7
Can begin to identify strengths and work with
them.
(Saleeby 1992)

5 Users'/clients' agenda   1–2–3–4–5–6–7
They should be in the driving seat as far as the
mandate will allow (this is usually more than we
generally estimate even when circumstances are
defined by a compulsory order).
(Marsh and Fisher 1992)

6 **Partnership**   1–2–3–4–5–6–7
Practice includes a task-centred approach –
deconstructs problems and reconstructs in
achievable bites – includes openness in recording
and written agreements.
(Doel and Marsh 1992)

7 **Process**   1–2–3–4–5–6–7
Can begin to see empowerment as a process and
believe people gain confidence and competence
(often) over a long time.
(Keiffer 1984)

8 **Transitions**   1–2–3–4–5–6–7
Have become skilled in working in 'mesosystems' –
between groups, *between* organisations, making
links.
(Bronfenbrenner 1979)

9 **Critical reflection**   0–1–2–3–4–5–6–7
Can begin to appreciate how users/clients might
examine some of the external origins to their
problems (without burdening them). This is
advanced practice and best achieved in groups.
(Freire 1972; Mullender and
Ward 1991; Reisch *et al.* 1981)

10 **Values**   1–2–3–4–5–6–7
Can understand the implication of having strongly
held values and have expectations of clients:
(a) mutual respect
(Cochran 1985)

11 **Values**   1–2–3–4–5–6–7
(b) anti-discrimination – gender, race/ethnicity,
disability, sexuality, age, etc.
(Macdonald 1991)

12 **Values**   1–2–3–4–5–6–7
(c) anti-violence – e.g. towards women, children,
elders, those with disabilities.
(Mullender and Ward 1991)

13 **Citizenship**   1–2–3–4–5–6–7
Can begin to understand the implications of
inclusiveness and participation as an expression
of citizenship.
(Keiffer 1984)

14 Cultural sensitivity   1–2–3–4–5–6–7
Acknowledge diversity and can begin to
understand users/clients in terms of their own
particular history and culture.
(Mullender and Ward 1991)

15 Rights   1–2–3–4–5–6–7
Believe in rights and can begin to assess factors
which may contribute to denial of rights.
(Cochran 1985)

16 And responsibilities   1–2–3–4–5–6–7
Can be seen to *have expectations* of people (e.g.
as parents) and to encourage responsibility.
(Bronfenbrenner 1987)

17 Challenge   1–2–3–4–5–6–7
Acknowledge that people need to be challenged.
This implies other roles – e.g. membership role in
a group, through work, or training, or education.
(Bronfenbrenner 1987)

18 Care   1–2–3–4–5–6–7
Appreciate that the empowerment process often
requires for people at least three kinds of
relationship – *being cared for*, actually as well as
in the sense of unconditional acceptance.
(Cochran 1985)

19 Group membership   1–2–3–4–5–6–7
Can begin to articulate what is needed to facilitate
directly or indirectly for users'/clients' *membership
of a group*.
(Cochran 1985, Mullender and Ward 1991)

20 A mentor   1–2–3–4–5–6–7
Can understand the value of the *mentor* role – an
individual who counsels, encourages, helps
client/user to sustain commitment to a course of
action – and can begin to articulate how to locate
such a person.
(Cochran 1985)

21 Staff empowerment   1–2–3–4–5–6–7
Can begin to consider how workers ought to be
empowered to work in this way.
(Parsloe and Stevenson 1993; Simon 1994)

REFERENCES

Adams, R. (1990) *Self-Help, Social Work and Empowerment*, London: Macmillan.

Barber, J. G. (1991) *Beyond Casework*, Basingstoke: Macmillan.

Barker, I. and Peck, E. (1987) *Power in Strange Places: User Empowerment in Mental Health Services*, London: Good Practices in Mental Health.

Berger, P. L. and Neuhaus, R. J. (1977) *To Empower People: the Role of Mediating Structures in Public Policy*, Washington DC: American Enterprise Institute for Public Policy Research.

Brechín, A., Liddiard, P. and Swain, J. (eds). (1981) *Handicap in a Social World*, London: Hodder & Stoughton/OUP Press.

Bronfenbrenner, U. (1979) *The Ecology of Human Behaviour*, Cambridge, MA: Harvard University Press.

Bronfenbrenner, U. (1987) 'Foreword. Family support: the quiet revolution', in Kagan, S., Powell, D. R., Weissbourd, B., Zigler, E. F. (eds), *America's Family Support Programs*, New Haven: Yale University Press, pp. xi–xvii.

Cammasso, M. J. and Cammasso, A. E. (1986) 'Social supports, undesirable life events, and psychological distress in a disadvantaged population', *Social Services Review*, September: 378–95.

Cochran, M. (1985) 'The parental empowerment process: building upon family strengths', in John Harris (ed.), *Child Psychology in Action: Linking Research and Practice*, London: Croom Helm.

Cochran, M. (1987) 'Empowering families: an alternative to the deficit model', in Hurrelman, K., Kaufman, F. X., Losel, F. (eds), *Social Interventions: Potential and Constraints*, Berlin: de Gruyter.

Cochran, M. and Brassard, J. (1979) 'Child development and personal social networks', *Child Development*, 50: 60, 601–16

Cochran, M. and Henderson, C. Jr (1990) 'Family supports and informal social ties: a case study', in Cochran M., Larner M., Riley D., Gunnarsson, L., and Henderson, C. Jr, *Extending Families: The Social Networks of Parents and their Children*, Cambridge/New York: Cambridge University Press.

Connolly, M. (1989) 'An act of empowerment: the Children, Young Persons and their Families Act', *British Journal of Social Work*, 24: 87–100.

Craig, G., Mayo, M. and Taylor, M. (1990) 'Empowerment: a continuing role for community development', *Community Development Journal*, 25 (4): 286–90.

DHSS (Department of Health and Social Security) (1985) *Social Work Decisions in Child Care – Recent Research Findings and their Implications*, London: HMSO.

DoH (Department of Health) (1992–5) 'The Family Support Initiative', evaluation by J. Hartless and C. Warren. Unpublished.

Doel, M. and Marsh, P. (1992) *Task Centred Social Work*, Aldershot: Ashgate Publishing Ltd.

Dunst, C. (1990) *Family Support Principles: Checklist for Program Builders and Practitioners: Family Systems Intervention Monograph, 2, No 5*, Morganton, NC: Family, Infant and Pre-School Program, Western Carolina Centre.

Dunst, C., Trivette, C. and Deal, A. (eds). (1994) *Supporting and Strengthening Families*, Cambridge, MA: Brookline Books.

Freeman, E., Logan S. and Gowdy E. (1992) 'Empowering single mothers', *Affilia*, 7 (2): 123–41.

Freire, P. (1972) *Pedagogy of the Oppressed*, Harmondsworth: Penguin.

Freynet, M.-F. (1995) *Les Médiations du Travail Social*, Lyon: Chroniques Sociales.

FRG (Family Rights Group) (1991) *The Children Act 1989: Working in Partnership with Families*, London: HMSO.

Gibbons, J. (ed.) (1992) *The Children Act 1989 and Family Support: Principles into Practice*, London: HMSO.

Goldberg, E. and Sinclair, I. (1986) *Family Support Exercises*, London: National Institute for Social Work.

Guttierrez, L.M. (1990) 'Working with women of color: an empowerment perspective', *Social Work*, 35: 149–502.

Hasenfield, Y. (1987) 'Power in social work practice', *Social Services Review*, September, 459–83.

Heger, R. L. and Hunzeker, J. M. (1988) 'Moving toward empowerment-based practice in public child welfare', *Social Work*, November/December: 499–502.

Holdsworth, L. (1991) *Empowerment Social Work With Physically Disabled People*, *Social Work Monographs*, University of East Anglia.

Howe, D. (1987) *An Introduction to Social Work Theory*, Aldershot: Wildwood House.

Kagan, S., Powell, D. R., Weissbourd, B. and Zigler, E. F. (eds). (1987) *America's Family Support Programs*, New Haven: Yale University Press.

Keiffer, C. H. (1984) 'Citizen empowerment: A developmental perspective', *Prevention in Human Services*, 3 (Winter/Spring): 9–36.

Macdonald, S. (1991) *All Equal Under The Act*, London: Race Equality Unit/National Institute for Social Work.

Maluccio, A., Fein, E. and Olmstead, K. (1986) *Permanency Planning for Children*, London/New York: Tavistock.

Marsh, P. and Fisher, M. (1992) *Good Intentions: Developing Partnership in Social Services*, York: Community Care/ Rowntree.

Mullender, A. and Ward, D. (1991) *Self-Directed Group-Work*, London: Whiting & Birch.

Parsloe, P. and Stevenson, O. (1993) *Community Care and Empowerment*, York: Community Care/ Rowntree.

Parsons, R. (1991) 'Empowerment: purpose and practice principle in social work', *Social Work with Groups*, 14 (2): 7–21.

Pinderhughes, E. (1983) 'Empowerment for our clients and ourselves', *Social Casework: Journal of Contemporary Social Work*, June: 331–8.

Rappoport, J. (1995) cited in Networking Bulletin from Cornell Empowerment project, G19A MVR Hall, Cornell University, Ithaca, NY 14853.

Reisch, M., Wenocur, S. and Sherman, W. (1981) 'Empowerment, conscientization and animation as core social work skills', *Social Development Issues*, 5 (2–3): 109–20.

Rose, W. (1992) 'Foreword', in Gibbons, J. (ed.) (1992) *The Children Act 1989 and Family Support: Principles into Practice*, London: HMSO.

Saleeby, D. (1992) *The Strengths Perspective in Social Work Practice*, New York: Longman.

Simon, B. L. (1990) 'Rethinking empowerment', *Journal of Progressive Human Services*, 1 (1): 27–39.

Simon, B. L. (1994) *The Empowerment Tradition in American Social Work*, NY/Chichester: Columbia University Press.

Solomon, B. (1987) 'Empowerment: social work in oppressed communities', *Journal of Social Work Practice*, May: 79–91.

Part II

New practices with children and families

Chapter 6

New social networks for families and children in Germany

Annemarie Gerzer-Sass and Rudolf Pettinger

EDITORS' INTRODUCTION

This chapter describes family self-help centres in Germany. Self-help traditionally has an important place in German social policy; while self-help organisations are as diverse in Germany as elsewhere, those described here have emerged from a movement of parents. This movement has its origins in the 1968 student revolt against rigid, uncreative norms and practices in the care and education (the German term pedagogy includes both these areas) of children and young people. In Chapter 4, Crescy Cannan refers to the parallel parents' movement in France.

Family self-help centres then introduce not just the principles of parent participation or self-management in a pluralistic welfare state, but challenge professional theories and empower parents. This chapter describes the ways in which lay and professional workers have been able to find ways of working together while becoming much more responsive to local needs. These are mainly for flexible day care for children, including those of school age, for opportunities for building social networks, for informal education, and for a child-friendly public environment. As in the UK, preventive family support lies at the centre of the recent (1990) Children and Young People Act, whose significance for the self-help movement is discussed.

FAMILIES CALL FOR SELF-HELP INITIATIVES

In West Germany in the last fifteen years something new has supplemented the traditional axis of family policy: families as receivers of family policy measures are speaking up for themselves in the founding of projects, for example: mother, family and neighbourhood centres, parents' initiatives, or mother and children groups.

These initiatives fit into a broader self-help movement in the health and psychosocial spheres. They are all expressions of a cultural change which – initiated by the 1968 student revolution – created, through a broad criticism of social institutions, a new kind of social-political action. Building on this were small, i.e. town or community-based, informal services operating in the area outside formal welfare organisations, leading to a separation between 'state help' and 'self-help' (Evers and Ostner 1989).

Family self-help initiatives used their connection to family life to work against the increasing separation between private and public domains through the creation of new self-determined neighbourly support and communication networks. In this way new connections were created for mothers between their private family work and their social and public life for which there have been few precedents.

Contrary to the so-called modernising logic, where self-determination and self-affirmation are made possible in the world of work dominated by individual achievement, we find the role of the mother which implies values such as continuing and reliable relationships, commitment, closeness and being there for each other. Everyone – regardless of gender – who engages with the logic of caring – experiences this contradiction, because the caring role is connected with an 'un-completed modernisation' concerning the distribution of opportunities, types of work and dependencies and therefore a real experienced disadvantage (cf. Beck 1985). It is still mainly women who leave gainful employment after the birth of their children; however, this is no longer a lifelong decision, but temporary, with the intention of re-entering the labour market.

Consequently the 'housewife' is not disappearing. Approximately half of all young women live as housewives as long as their children are small, although there is increasing employment of women with young children. During the last twenty years the number of mothers with children under the age of 6 in gainful employment has increased from 33 to 39 per cent. Interesting changes have occurred. In the past the status of housewife was a social privilege and a proof of the earning power of the husband. This picture has changed; now women who opt for a longer period as a housewife are an underprivileged group with regard to their education and opportunities in the labour market (Erler *et al.* 1988: 11).

The situation was completely different in East Germany where more than 90 per cent of women worked until unification. Full-time gainful employment of women was part of their state-decreed 'normal biography' which left no room for individually creating roles, especially alternative roles as housewives, or working significantly shorter hours because of family commitments. These alternatives were officially not catered for with resulting ideological and material discrimination (Jaeckel 1990: 47). Today we see a certain return to traditional roles because it is mainly women who are affected by the transformation of the labour market. This means that we can assume almost a 50 per cent reduction in the gainful employment of women with small children (Bertram *et al.* 1994: 53).

All these women, whether they live in East or West Germany, experience the structural conflict 'of the unfinished modernisation of the role of mother' and its connected 'non-conformism to modernity'; it can be felt as a personal dilemma; the role of mother is experienced as a failure, lack of ability and low self-esteem.

To 'solve' this structural conflict strategies are developed which almost exclusively aim at including women in the employment world in spite of their family work, letting them take part in 'the rules of modernity' in that way. Public initiatives such as, for example, professional training for women and parents, do not really engage with the structural dilemma in which most mothers find themselves. This kind of training offers mostly advice for the 'self-improvement' of mothers, implying that the *role of mother* needs improvement.

The concept of the family self-help initiatives, especially the mother and family centres points in an opposite direction. They offer the social novelty of a child-friendly, interested public environment where neither change nor conformity is demanded from the mothers. They do not have to adapt their children to child-hostile norms to gain at least some public acceptance as mothers, nor do they have to 'free' themselves from their children to be respected as adult women. The idea is based on women's demand to have a more public life with children as well as notable opposition arising from two aspects of life: on the one hand the isolated everyday life of the nuclear family and on the other hand everyday employment life mainly orientated to male biographies (cf. Gerzer-Sass 1991).

Therefore family self-help's own understanding is based neither on a description of families' deficiencies nor on an overcoming of the family but is orientated to its own resources and thus its capacity for renewal. The movement seeks to address both individual psychosocial needs and those of the family without wanting to diminish or supersede the family and its relations (cf. Tüllmann and Erler 1988: 316ff.).

MOTHER, FAMILY AND NEIGHBOURHOOD CENTRES: THE DOMAIN OF FAMILY SELF-HELP

The family self-help movement takes part in making public life favourable for families and children. There are now about 340 self-help family centres in Germany. Unlike the family centres of the big, formal welfare organisations (notably Caritas (the Catholic church), Diakonie (the Protestant church) and Arbeiterwohlfahrt (linked with the Social Democratic Party)) self-help family centres do not rely on professionals' work. Instead they emerge from people's own needs and empower people to create their own forms of help.

These centres adapt their structures to children's needs and the family time rhythm, perceiving children as part of adult culture. This is expressed in the buildings, the opening hours, the facilities, the furnishings and the emotional climate. Children have their own rooms and activities, but can also join in the activities and the life of the adults, giving them something like the experience of an extended family. Specific features of a centre are:

- regular advice and open access: mother-and-children cafés, sales of second-hand children's clothing, social services help and contact points for specific situations, for example, single parents;
- self-organised, lay help in the neighbourhood, accessible because based on the everyday experience of families. The ground rule is that everybody has abilities which he or she can share at the centre. This is true for the old and the young and in different phases of life and for different interests. The self-help principle makes democratic participation in the organisation and in its decision-making process possible;
- despite the self-help principle, regular and contracted work at the centre is paid on a fixed hourly rate. This funding, as for other centre costs, usually comes from the city or community council – once the group has persuaded the council of the value of their work. This appeals to women who would otherwise have difficulties getting involved for financial, social or time reasons.

A further important conceptual basis is related to the 'open' child care in the mother and family centres. This is seen as a complementary and additional service to the child care services of the formal welfare organisations. It is a challenge to them as was shown in the research and development programme of model projects in which the authors were engaged: 'A place for children' (Arbeitsgruppe 'Orte für Kinder' 1995). This showed that an effective model for care is a supplement to crèche, nursery school or day care centre because it suits the different needs of mothers as well as fulfilling children's pedagogical needs. Given changes in family structures and the one-child family, children particularly need broader social learning experiences. This child care model

- complements institutional care because it is flexible, hourly and not necessarily regular; it does not require complex application and registration procedures: this pattern does not exist in ordinary day care establishments;
- supplements other arrangements. In the centres children of different ages and from different backgrounds can, over shorter or longer periods of time, gain experiences beyond their family, not only with each other but also with their own mothers and with other adults. Human interrelationships rather than pedagogical considerations rule the children's world: children experience public life as communal life where they can learn consideration for each other, capacity for understanding and an experience of time;
- challenges the structured 'pedagogised' everyday life of children. At the same time it is a challenge to the profession of child care staff because in the centres the mothers not only look after their own children but look after the children of other women as well.

The impact of these concepts lies on different levels:

The socially preventative character of family self-help – overcoming privatisation and individualisation

In the preventive sense of family welfare, family centres help cope with the continuous need to adapt and learn in the family. The non-treatment character of the centres enables women to exchange the worries, problems, conflicts and needs of 'normal' family life, to receive or give advice, and to learn from the experiences of others. This form of public life enables the majority of families, by considering other family situations, to recognise and work out structural conflicts and problems which otherwise would have been seen and treated as self-inflicted. Although the private sphere is always respected, the privacy of the family is no longer taboo. The preventive character of the family self-help centres makes another taboo, domestic violence, easier to talk about.

The preventive character of the centres has its limits: there are always women who are looking for and are in need of professional advice or therapeutic help for themseves or their families. Here the centres can help with finding contacts with the appropriate services as well as encouraging the women to approach them.

The centres have not developed into meeting points for 'frustrated housewives' – as had been feared by lots of husbands who imagined that their women, supported by the centres, would turn against them. Instead they have become places where women can think about their relationships with their partners. The centres initiate the development of new networks, in which the men can also be integrated, participating as 'good neighbours'. In this way the stability of the family is supported and the relationship between partners relieved and enriched.

Opportunities for public participation of mothers

The centres have proved themselves to be places where mothers can participate in society as well as getting help in integrating into employment and public life. The motto 'everybody is capable of something' encourages everyone. Age, education and job training are less important than family life experiences. Through self-determined learning, identity and self-confidence are strengthened. With their help, over one-third of the women have been able to return to work or increase their commitment to public life or social service in the community.

It has been found however, that it is impossible or very difficult to gain regular financial support for this kind of informal learning, education or further education because it does not correspond with the conditions for publicly supported programmes for people returning to work or for adult education. A significant hindrance is the requirement for professional qualifications; unqualified teachers are not accepted. Questions about efficiency and quality are often only answered according to formal criteria. Abilities and qualities such as love, the ability to form relationships, listening to each other, solidarity, etc., which originate in the area of family life, are not accepted criteria. But these values and abilities are especially significant for the further development of their own personality and the personal success of many women.

This does not mean that professional work and education is superfluous or could or should be substituted by unqualified or voluntary workers. But experiences in family and neighbourhood centres have shown that with corresponding financial support a higher quality can be achieved by these lay workers than in some services of adult education and job training. It is therefore necessary to re-think the terms of qualification and education on which the public social services are based and to integrate initiatives and experience from the area of family self-help into existing and future programmes. This way it would not only enrich the existing education landscape but would provide an opportunity for a great number of women who fall through the net of public programmes because of their commitment to their families over a shorter or longer period of time.

The activities of family self-help have proved, then, to be an important help in integrating family women into jobs and public life. It is important that this group of women should take the opportunity to gain qualifications, but criteria of qualifications should be measured less by the logic of the world of employment and more by the skills the women have gained within the framework of family life or family self-help.

Child-friendly public life

Children are part of the public life of the centre but not its focus. They are not seen as a disturbing factor in adults' groups nor as a group which has to be cared for; rather they are seen as a part of public group experience, in which there is room for other dimensions such as consideration, sympathy and experience of time. Therefore a child-friendly environment is needed regarding rooms, opening hours, equipment and emotional climate.

This form of child-friendly public life has proved to be a main factor in relieving the strain for families. To participate in a child-friendly environment, structures are necessary which enable parents/mothers to act from the immediacy of their own experience. They know from their life with a child where improvements in their area of town or village are necessary, for example in

- more participation in town and traffic planning;
- continual co-operation between professional and lay (unqualified, user) knowledge; and
- the acceptance and support of family self-help child care as an important supplement to formal day care services.

For children under 3 years old there are only crèche places besides private arrangements. Existing places, though, in no way meet the demand for daily full-time child care outside the home for working mothers. The three-year extended parental leave has increased the demand for open, flexible child care arrangements for this age group (cf. Erler *et al.* 1988: 62). Often the family and neighbourhood centres help out with child care bottlenecks, for example with the lack of nursery school places, because they can react more spontaneously and less bureaucratically. In this way they integrate, for example children of nursery school age, until they get a nursery school place.

Stimulating a neighbourhood culture through voluntary and paid work

The creation of adequate living space for mothers and children (and also for special groups such as single parents and the elderly) is not a private matter, but a community task which should be as much a matter of course as building sports centres, swimming pools or car parks. It has been shown that the creation of family and neighbourhood centres means that not only families with their specific needs are catered for but that the quality of life in the whole community is enriched. Furthermore, the limitations of professional services for families and the neighbourhood become obvious, leading to new initiatives.

Such successes and achievements would not be possible without voluntary work as well as paid work. In future there will therefore be an increasing discussion about the boundaries between them, between professional work and unpaid work by mothers.

Paying lay or voluntary work does not necessarily damage the character of self-help. It is not a contradiction in terms. As long as the basic rules for family self-help are guaranteed by the state and funding agencies the innovative characteristics of this new social structure can be preserved. The more creative participation remains possible, the more opportunities for development remain open to all. The less professional systems and administration hinder the participation of volunteers, the more family self-help projects can preserve their specific features alongside the traditional welfare organisations. Otherwise these latter will sooner or later replace them, drive them out or take them over (Gerzer-Sass and Pettinger 1991).

Family self-help is therefore moving away from current ideas about prevention, which start with responding to individual parental mistakes in the upbringing of their children. Family self-help movements stand next to empowerment movements which aim at creating political pro-grammes and measures to enable people to receive and form the resources that impinge on their lives (Rappaport 1987: 269). The concept of empowerment initiates new ideas for the whole field of social work and social policy. The image of clients, stuck in self-blame or blame from others for their inadequacy and the need for help (still the prime legitimation of social work and its services), is confronted with the strength of the person. The receiver of social services is perceived as a competent actor, as a builder of a successful everyday life.

FAMILY SELF-HELP AND ITS INTEGRATION INTO THE WELFARE STATE: THE NEW CHILDREN AND YOUTH ACT

The expansion of social services through professional social work has been increasing over the last few years. The 1990 Children and Youth Support Act – the *Kinder- und Jugendhilfegesetz* or KJHG – with its extension, or rather its first legally binding provision, of services for children, young people and families, is going to increase this even further. This is especially true for preventive services (e.g. advice services), although these have to operate within very tight budgets due to the limited ways in which public money intended for social causes is distributed. With the increase of professional social services, there has been an increased interest in family self-help; the new law, implemented in 1991, specifically mentions self-help among the individual services. Day care of children (Section 25) and the general promotion of upbringing in the family can be supplied by self-help or neighbourhood centres and by associations of parents. There is an improvement in the legal basis for the support of self-help initiatives because of the general intentions of the law. This is seen in

• the strong emphasis on the preventive character of youth and family support;
• the stress on the family as the main place for children's socialisation, the priority of parents' responsibility in bringing up children and the duty under the KJHG law to support parents with this task.

Social prevention can be understood in another, social structural sense: the overall development of society. The changes in family structures underlie the need for, at least at certain developmental stages, help in socialisation. Prevention in this sense means the improvement in the quality of life through the construction of a social infrastructure for families and children (cf. Hebenstreit-Müller and Pettinger 1991: 165ff.). There is an underlying concept then, which is wider than that under the KJHG, where services are only for certain family situations and problems (for example, single parents or separation and divorce). So far there is no experience of the implementation of this statutorily supported family self-help; it will depend a lot on the (still awaited) individual state regulations (Germany is a federal state – eds.).

Family self-help produces a richer life compared with bigger, formal, welfare organisations because it is dependent on small solidarity networks and because it is more 'alive' through the building of small, easily comprehensible forms. Therefore family self-help questions the institutional structures of these big associations which are characterised by complex legal rules, rigid training regulations and their hierarchical set up. The pluralism principle in German social policy and the need for more choice in services mean that self-help measures complement the large, formal welfare providers.

Because of this, the relationship between professional social services and family self-help is often seen as competitive. The reason for this is mainly the fact that self-help arrangements work at much lower cost than professional services. This comparison, however, misses the fact that they deal with non-comparable tasks in care and education. The child care in mother and family centres aims at enabling contacts within and across age groups and at providing occasional respite for the parents, but not at care based on regularity and long-term learning and developmental concepts.

Self-help establishments and projects that offer child care as an alternative to crèches, nursery schools or day care centres are subject to the same personnel and qualification regulations as professional institutions if they are to receive public financial aid. Under these conditions the cost of family self-help is not very different from that of formal welfare organisations. The main differences between similar care arrangements at self-help and ordinary establishments lie in the possibilities of participation by the parents: in self-help centres a wide-ranging and responsible participation of parents is not only welcome but often required. It is the professional child care staff's duty to involve parents in the child care work. In formal organisations, however, the participation of the parents is precisely and legally prescribed, for example in representation in organisation management or in questions about the rights of parents. The routine participation of parents in child care is neither catered for nor legally possible.

Self-help centres and professional social services are based on different ideas of human beings: ideally, the first assume active, competent and self-responsible parents. The relationship between the parents is governed by the democratic principle of the same rights and the same duties. In formal organisations a principally hierarchical relationship exists between the qualified staff and the parents (laypeople) regarding the rules about competence and responsibility; the parents are granted competence in bringing up their children within the family – they do not get the chance to try and develop their abilities in a framework outside the family.

While the institutional child care services encourage a division of the child's world into separate spheres (family and day care are experienced as separate areas, behaviour varies between them), the self-help facilities try to maintain the unity of the child's world – through other forms of relationships and through the routine participation of parents. Participation and democratic relationships in the self-help centres often lead to this being transferred to other situations and encourage social responsibility and political participation, for example in the local community. The effects can be seen in changes in the opinions and self-confidence of the initiators of and participants in self-help projects.

Summing up, we argue that the view that the self-help services should or do substitute for professional services and institutions is only partially valid. It has to be said, though, that the conditions for public funding force the self-help measures to adopt professional standards (for example, the employment of qualified child care workers). The self-help character shows mainly in the participative structures of the centres, as well as in the behaviour between qualified staff and parents. But, in the main, child-oriented self-help services cover other family needs than those covered by the professional services. They supplement them, relieving parents at certain times and opening up and enriching their social and interpersonal lives.

NEW SOCIAL NETWORKS THROUGH A COMBINATION OF FAMILY SELF-HELP AND FORMAL WELFARE ORGANISATIONS: AN EXAMPLE FROM DAY CARE FOR CHILDREN

That formal organisations and family self-help should be brought together to co-operate rather than compete seems a good idea because the old welfare mixture is in need of reform. The example of established day care services shows how far today's welfare organisations are from the real needs of the parents and their children. Changes are necessary if they want to keep up with developments in society. As we have shown, their direction should be

* more flexible, sometimes hourly child care services;
* more democratic and less hierarchical structures which encourage grassroots involvement of parents, and increase the creativity and motivation of child care staff;
* more local opportunities to meet, where parents with children are wanted and are part of a public culture;
* more child care arrangements with a mix of ages up to 12 because this

gives children a broader experience of social learning and growing up and helps one-child families.

Such changes also mean new departures from established pedagogical theories. There should be

• a less structured daily life because the day care centre has to compensate for the unsuitability of children's living spaces due to child-hostile town planning and housing. Children also spend much longer in these centres than before, so they have to offer more scope for play and new experiences;
• pedagogical services that pick up on the movement of the 1970s which opposed cognitively oriented pre-school care and education. This approach originated in the '*Kinderladen*' movement (a co-operative movement of parents, setting up something like playgroups, associated with1968 – eds). These practised a so-called everyday life pedagogy. The children do what they would experience and do at home, for example, they go shopping, cook, etc. The principle of experiencing everyday life with children demands a degree of sensitivity to the world of children and a great emotional readiness to adapt to children and their needs. The subject-dominated training of child care staff falls short of these ideals, if they are conveyed at all.

Within our model project, 'A Place for Children', an attempt was made to combine the care initiatives of family self-help with formal welfare organisations' services, to create new social networks for families and their children. The function of models is to respond to social trends, and also to demonstrate a piece of social innovation which would not otherwise emerge due to established structures. Two places were chosen for the model projects which – although they had very different structures and entry conditions – were able to expand services due to close co-operation between the welfare organisations and family self-help.

One was a mothers' centre, established for ten years, offering a day care service like those of the formal welfare organisations. Once it looked at family needs, it widened its services to offer mixed-age, flexible and regular child care for children between 1 and 14 for local families. The specific approach of family self-help, as well as a self-managed structure and openness to the neighbourhood, was incorporated. Only the principle of qualified workers was broken, i.e. now mothers untrained in child care work alongside professional staff within the team of carers.

A family self-help group was integrated into a large institutional care centre with over 200 children. This improved the care services through additional flexible and hourly care. It also improved the centre by setting up a cafeteria area, a shop for second-hand children's clothing etc. so that it became a meeting place for parents with children in the centre and for families from the local community. The centre meant that some of the divisions in the community – between middle-class families and those in council housing – were moderated: people shared something beyond class and age. It became a very accessible centre, partly because it made it easy to move from looking for second-hand clothes, to having a coffee, to participating in the centre. Mothers and professional staff worked together.

The social and political volatility of co-operation between unqualified or voluntary workers and professionals, or rather the conflict between the logics of self-help and of organisations, lies mainly in the fact that the occupational image of child care staff is connected to the image of the loving substitute mother. In trying to gain professional status and better pay, child care staff try to escape from the socially inferior role of the mother. It was not the aim of the model projects to encourage child care workers' fears that mothers would question their professionalism and worsen their financial situation. Rather it was to encourage a mixture of different abilities: on the one hand the specialised abilities of the professional staff and on the other hand mothers' practical abilities and experience. Many mothers in nuclear families have built networks for themselves and their children, and become practical experts in community work – as is illustrated by the various initiatives in the area of family self-help.

The co-operation in the care centre described above was supported by a pedagogical theory in which caring, communal feeling and especially living together are at the centre. The laypeople learnt from the professionals (e.g. in the area of developmental psychology or teaching methods) and the professionals learnt from the mothers (e.g. flexibility and teamwork). The child care staff came to see co-operation with the laypeople as not only a supplement to their pedagogical work but as an improvement in the quality of care. They also felt more secure in being flexible about time and in their treatment of parents and other adults. However, it has needed the inclusion of mothers to enable child care centres to become more open to the neighbourhood. The centre has since developed into a lively neighbourhood centre.

FAMILY SELF-HELP IN EAST GERMANY

Until unification, family self-help activities were unheard of in East Germany. On the one hand, self-organised and self-determined initiatives were not politically encouraged, on the other hand there was no need because nearly all women were gainfully employed and child care was comprehensively organised. After unification the idea of family self-help – supported by West German initiatives – has been developed in East Germany as well. Now there are nearly thirty mothers' centres in East Germany.

The main reason for getting involved in family self-help was to help women cope with the changes better, by exchanging with others and influencing one's life as much as possible under the given circumstances. The centres have developed into spaces that mitigate against the increasing isolation of women who do not see opportunities for themselves on the labour market any more or who had become unemployed. But they have also developed into meeting places for an increasing number of mothers who have deliberately chosen a longer period of parental leave.

Because of the dramatic reduction in the number of births – since unification the number of births has halved within two years (Fünfter Familienbericht (Fifth Family Report of the Ministry for Families and Elderly People)1994: 36) – the mothers' centres have proved to be a useful meeting place for other groups in society. A deliberate attempt has been made to involve older women and men, who are often unemployed, in the everyday life of the centres. As first investigations show, the centres are not only contributing to stabilising the situation of the women involved but also activating hidden resources for communal life. But these are only in single initiatives which, in view of the desperately needed social infrastructure, cannot cover the need for advice, support and help for families.

The self-help projects in the new states were set up under West German conditions and regulations, for example according to criteria for state-aided job creation or support projects. After initial problems they are gradually finding their own identity. The basic problem was, and still is, the fact that professionalism, or rather paid work, has a high status in the new states and that therefore combinations of paid, professional and lay, voluntary work and competence are very hard to implement.

CONCLUSION

The development of family self-help in East and West Germany has one point in common: in neither area does it fit into the traditional structure of social services. Its identity means crossing boundaries and going in new directions.

First, family self-help practises new forms of work because voluntary work is – in self-help practice – paid for at a fixed rate. In this way unconventional work relationships, through a mixture of professional and lay knowledge, have been developed. Second, the question of how we judge the quality of child care is raised; up to now it has been measured by the qualifications of the staff. Third, new forms of relationship question the social service professions' ideal of distance in professional attitudes.

New forms of work in the public sector still fall under traditional regulations. The public sector has never seriously considered the transfer of social competences and qualifications that have been acquired and developed within the framework of family life to other public areas (one exception is home-economics training). A fundamental debate about new demands of the labour market is needed to start this transfer. These demands are for qualities that can only partly be acquired through school or formal training. The new welfare mix will contribute to a new definition of professionalism, which increasingly will have to be defined more through social experience than formally acquired expertise.

In this new form of welfare pluralism traditional actors – like the state, the market (firms), welfare organisations – would have to deal with a new partner, namely the family. If the family were accepted as a serious partner in this co-operation, it would question the established time structures, professional knowledge and hierarchies of the existing welfare partners.

So far the family has not had a chance against the dominance and logic of the other institutions. Maybe the 'in between' level of the self-help organisations will enable the family to become a more powerful partner in future co-operation, especially as self-help structures are nearer to the users than the welfare state. In this way self-help can not only start the empowerment process on an individual level but can also resist the structural lack of consideration in relation to families (Fünfter Familienbericht 1994). The model is still too young to judge finally whether self-help structures can – in co-operation with them – change public institutions in the long term. The future, however, will depend on more mixtures in welfare state programmes to sharpen the sense of a welfare state pluralism responding to changing social needs.

REFERENCES

Arbeitsgruppe 'Orte für Kinder' (1995), unpublished final report of the model project *Orte für Kinder* (A Place for Children) for the Federal Ministry for the Family, Senior Citizens, Women and Youth, Deutsches Jugendinstitut (German Youth Institute), München.

Beck, U. (1985) *Risikogesellschaft, Auf den Weg in eine andere Moderne*, Frankfurt/Main: Suhrkamp.

Bertram, B., Erler, G., Jaeckel, M. and Sass, J. (1994) 'Auswirkungen und Einschätzungen familienpolitischer Maßnahmen für Familien mit Kindern unter 6 Jahren im europäischen Vergleich' (Consequences and Evaluations of European Family Policies for Families and Children under 6 years of Age in the European Union), unpublished research report, Deutsches Jugendinstitut, München.

Erler, G., Jaeckel, M., Pettinger, R. and Sass, J. (1988) *Kind? Beruf? oder beides?*, Hamburg: Brigitte Untersuchung 88.

Evers, A. and Ostner, I. (1989) 'Arbeit und Engagement im intermediären Bereich', *Beiträge zur Sozialpolitik*, Köln: Forschung, Bd.4.

Fünfter Familienbericht (Fifth Family Report) (1994) *Familien und Familienpolitik im geeinten Deutschland – Zukunft des Humanvermögens'* (Families and Family Policy in Unified Germany – Future of Human Ability), Federal Ministry for Families and Senior Citizens, Bonn

Gerzer-Sass, A. (1991) 'Qualifizierung von Müttern', in S. Hebenstreit-Müller and R. Pettinger (eds), *Miteinander lernen, leben, engagieren – Neue soziale Netze für Familien*, Theorie und Praxis der Frauenforschung, vol.15, Bielefeld: Kleine.

Gerzer-Sass, A. and Pettinger, R. (1991) *Wo Familien selbst aktiv sind! Erfahrungen aus dem Modellprojekt Familien helfen Familien*, Nürnberg: EAF Bayern.

Gerzer-Sass, A. and Pettinger, R. (1993) 'Kinderbetreuung in Selbsthilfe', in J. Becker-Textor and M. Textor (eds) *Handbuch der Kinder und Jugendbetreuung*, Neuwied: Luchterhand.

Hebenstreit-Müller, S. and Pettinger, R. (eds) (1991) *Miteinander lernen, leben, engagieren – Neue soziale Netze für Familien*, Bielefeld: Kleine.

Jaeckel, M. (1990) 'Länderbericht DDR', in 'Familienpolitik im Umbruch? Ergebnisse einer explorativen Studie zu familienpolitschen Maßnahmen in der DDR, Polen, Sowjetunion und Ungarn', unpublished research report, Arbeitsgruppe Familienpolitik (Family Policy Working Group), Deutsches Jugendinstitut, München.

Rappaport, J. (1987) 'Terms of empowerment/exemplar of prevention: towards a theory for community psychology', *American Journal of Community Psychology*, 15 (2): 121–8.

Tüllmann, G. and Erler, G. (1988) 'Familienselbsthilfe – Ein neues Konzept stellt sich vor', in Deutsches Jugendinstitut (ed.) *Wie gehts der Familie? Ein Handbuch zur Situation der Familien heute*, München: Kösel.

Chapter 7

The role of the centre in family support

Eva Lloyd

VALUES AND OBJECTIVES OF SAVE THE CHILDREN'S CENTRE-BASED FAMILY SUPPORT

Save the Children's centre-based family support offers part-time and full-time day care, holiday playschemes, out-of-school, and community health services for children, and welfare rights advice, education and training for other members of their families, as well as self-help opportunities to develop a variety of groups, credit unions and food co-ops, and some youth work. It operates in this way from fifteen multi-functional centres located in some of the most deprived communities in the UK. These are staffed primarily by workers with a background in child care, youth and community work, and community development, run, if not managed, in partnership with centre users and funded through partnerships with a range of statutory agencies, including health, social services and education.

While Warren (1993: 5) has claimed that 'The bedeviling feature of family centres has been a lack of definition', Save the Children centres have been well defined by Long (1995) as follows, in a discussion of their role in ameliorating family poverty:

> Save the Children centres are not to be viewed within the 'crisis oriented' model of interventions which offer 'therapeutic' help to families and children in need, but are firmly based within the community development framework. They provide practical responses to locally defined need. The principles of open access, self referral and user participation are fundamental to this approach. The anti-poverty strategy which underpins this work has two themes. The services seek to provide 'better beginnings' for children and 'new opportunities' for adults.
>
> (Long 1995: 64)

This chapter focuses on 'better beginnings' for children and on the implications of the current UK social policy context for Save the Children's centre-based family support, as seen from a management perspective. It is based on a 1993 review of this work conducted by the author.

The term family support is used here with reference to the Children Act 1989 and its associated Guidance, where family centres are identified 'as having a part to play in a continuum of family support services' (Warren 1993: 10). It has been defined by the Audit Commission (1994) as an activity or facility aimed at providing advice and support to parents to help them in bringing up their children. While the term 'family centre' will also be employed, centre-based family support is used in preference to denote the particular emphasis within Save the Children's work in this area.

Using Hardiker *et al.*'s (1995) framework for analysing services of this kind, Save the Children's model of provision reflects a welfare approach which combats social disadvantage by targeting a first level of prevention for populations and vulnerable communities. In this approach social inequality is perceived to lie at the root of social problems, including child abuse.

In these centres the strong influence of community development methods of working identified by Cannan (1992) on the type of family support provided, results from a commitment to

enabling people living in poor communities to participate in projects, and to increasing the strengths of such communities by enhancing the capabilities of individuals to enter into reciprocal exchanges – the basis of a social network.

(Cannan 1992: 105)

This commitment has its roots in the rights based approach taken by Save the Children from the start in all its work with children and their families in communities around the world.

A charter of Rights of the Child was developed by its founder Eglantyne Jebb in 1923 and adopted by the League of Nations in 1924. It can still be recognised in the 1989 United Nations Convention on the Rights of the Child, ratified by the UK government in 1991, which now guides the agency's work.

OPPORTUNITIES AND CHALLENGES FOR FAMILY SUPPORT

In the middle of the 1990s Save the Children centres find themselves at a crossroads. One the one hand a clear message is coming through from the Children Act 1989 (Department of Health 1991; Gibbons 1992), from recent research (Gibbons 1990; Smith 1993) and from central government's public services watchdog the Audit Commission (1994), that the open access and non-stigmatising model of family support delivered by Save the Children is preferable to services geared more exclusively to children at risk of significant harm.

On the other hand the rapidly changing policy context in which children's services are being delivered mitigates against this approach. The current local authority emphasis is on targeting children as dictated by the 'in need' definition employed in the Children Act 1989, for what are essentially child protection services. These are delivered mainly on the basis of service-level contracts agreed with voluntary-sector or independent agencies.

The Community Care Act 1990 introduced the market place to the delivery of services that traditionally had been the responsibility of local government. This model of service delivery has since been extended from health to personal social services, and children's services plans have been made mandatory. That the contract culture represents an appropriate model for the organisation of children's services remains in doubt, however (Jones and Bilton 1994).

As far as the impact of these developments on centre-based family support provision is concerned, 'There is little evidence of research, or even discussion of the role of family centres within the new context of the welfare market place' (Warren 1993: 10).

At the same time local government has been going through one of the most far-reaching reorganisations ever of both its format and its function. While these changes are taking place, developments in education, such as the introduction of local management for schools, the move towards grant-maintained schools, and currently the nursery-vouchers initiative, cut right across policy and practice supported by social services and health and contribute to growing inequality (Smith and Noble 1995).

These developments cannot easily be reconciled with the creation of a more integrated system of support for families with young children, bringing together health, education and social services. This kind of integrated support (which can be found in a number of Save the Children centres working in partnership with local health and other agencies) is recommended by policy analysts (Pugh 1992; Pugh and McQuail 1995; Cohen and Fraser 1991; Holtermann 1995a) and by the Children Act 1989 itself.

Although voluntary sector, or not-for-profit agencies obviously have an important role to play in the new services set-up, another role they traditionally fulfilled is being jeopardised. This is the opportunity their dual-funding base of voluntary income, coupled with block grants from statutory sources, gave them to innovate, to experiment, and to produce new models of service delivery. Such models were often 'mainstreamed', i.e. were taken over by the statutory agencies, or their characteristics were widely copied as good practice.

(This freedom to manoeuvre is being curtailed not only by the contract culture, but also by a steady fall in their voluntary income, which is due to a number of factors, the introduction of the National Lottery in 1994 being one.)

Service-level contracts for the delivery of services that arise from local government duties under the Children Act may not match the aspirations of or reflect need as perceived by the voluntary child care sector. This applies to the intake and management of family support centres as much as to other services for children and families.

(The third major challenge of the 1990s facing agencies such as Save the Children in the UK is a spectacular rise in levels of un- employment, and of child and family poverty)(Bradshaw 1992; Kumar 1993; Oppenheim 1994; Barclay 1995).

(Against this background, the major issues for Save the Children's centre-based family support work highlighted by the 1993 review (Lloyd 1993) were: issues around sustaining a universalist model of family support, around protecting its non-stigmatising character by retaining a balance between protection and support in favour of the latter, around determining the optimal balance between service delivery and advocacy in this area, and around attracting both public and private finance to fund these developments.)

(The resolution of these issues has become particularly acute for Save the Children as the result of a funding crisis in 1996. This has some of its origins in an inability to increase current levels of voluntary income and in the fact that the models of provision it operates with both in the UK and abroad do not easily attract the type of statutory funding now available. This is ironic in the light of the evidence, summarised below, that its approach to centre-based family support addresses all the factors recently identified by policy analysts, including the government's own, as important and relevant. If the current crisis is not speedily resolved, this chapter could become an epitaph for provision increasingly seen to be needed by young children and their families.)

THE ORIGINS OF SAVE THE CHILDREN'S CENTRE MODEL

The origins of Save the Children's model of centre-based family support were different from those of other child care agencies, which may explain its nature and the direction it took. The majority of centres emerged from single or amalgamated playgroups run in poor urban areas in the 1970s and 1980s. Their development was paralleled by the emergence of different species of family centre in other parts of the county (Walker 1991).

As a result of the Save the Children groups providing for some of the mothers' own needs as well as for those of their children, they success-fully attracted the more disadvantaged families. Playgroups requiring more intensive mother participation were failing to reach them, according to research by Joseph and Parfitt (1972), Ferri and Niblett (1977) and Finch (1983), reviewed by Lloyd et al. (1989).

By responding to the range and extent of the needs identified in these communities, Save the Children transformed the playgroups into multi functional resource centres, providing a kind of help to children and parents that 'most playgroups are not equipped to provide' (Ferri and Niblett 1977: 72). Quite early on, these centres had already come to be associated with the goals of prevention in the widest sense (Jackson 1986).

Centre staff perceived a relationship between community character-istics and families' childrearing and other practical problems and de-veloped methods to tackle these in partnership with centre users. Recently, this approach has received increasing attention, especially in the United States (Earls et al. 1994; Garbarino and Kostelny 1992).

In an analysis of the role of family centres, Smith (1993) identified four different debates which can serve as a route towards understanding their development:

> The current interest in family centres is most clearly rooted in the third and fourth of these debates – that is, in debates about 'prevention', 'at risk', 'need' and 'disadvantage', intervention and effectiveness. But the first and second debates, about education and care, and social networks and participation, are also important. The question is not only how such projects can help directly with children already in dif-ficulties, but also how they can influence the 'educational climate' of the home and the neighbourhood and the social networks which are the supportive fabric of the community.
>
> (Smith 1993: 16)

Save the Children centres combine all these approaches in various permutations. Arguably this is both their strength and their weakness in the current policy and funding climate.

DISTINGUISHING FEATURES

By the early 1990s Save the Children centres were not only operating outreach work with, for instance, West African and Vietnamese families and 'satellite' services such as support for child minders, but were often effectively at the disposal of communities for seven days a week, offering opportunities for autonomous activities organised by local groups, such as community playgroups, women's and girls' groups, credit unions and language classes.

> The centres encourage and support parents to set up new ventures out in the community, as well as within the centre itself. . . . In this sense, the centres are not just buildings where services are provided, but projects where workers enable other groups to make provision for themselves.
>
> (Statham 1994: 27)

This role for users in deciding what sort of provision best meets their needs is identified by Statham as a particular form of community development which strengthens the community base of these centres and fosters the local community perception of them as a community resource.

The Save the Children model of centre-based family support combines features characteristic of family centres studied by Holman (1988) and by De'Ath (1988). The client-focused, neighbourhood and community development models they described developed during the same period as the Save the Children models, which also share features of the seven types Warren (1991) distinguished between in his family centre typology.

While partnerships with users in the running and sometimes in the management of the centres characterise all centre-based family support, the 1993 management review highlighted that it displays certain paradoxical features. Sometimes Save the Children support is conceived of by managers as aiming towards community ownership of the facility, while at other times the security of long-term funding, which may only be available if voluntary or statutory agencies are involved, may be seen as the determinant of successful user participation.

It is a fact that long-term funding for community projects constitutes a problem for all centres of this kind as well as for other types of provision (Williams 1993), irrespective of the handover policy operated by senior management. It is also a fact that centres such as these are unlikely to be taken over by the community while this remains without its own resources.

The centres' open-access community-based approach is based on the key principles of the offer of a variety of provision, flexibility and responsiveness, lack of stigma, participation of users, and the provision of high-quality and affordable day care, while taking into account the social, gender and cultural factors affecting its users. Open access in this context means that the provision is in principle open to all, although demand entails that in practice all centres have had to develop priority admission policies.

Many do cater for children recognised as 'in need' under the Children Act, such as children with disabilities or on the 'at risk' register. Their broad range of users are predominantly united by poverty, and include a substantial proportion of female-headed single-parent families. The centres operate mostly integrated but occasionally specialist facilities, combining 'a remedial and preventive approach' (Statham 1994: 13).

Rarely, though, does this involve the therapeutic interventions encountered in some other statutory or voluntary family centres. Some centres reserve places for referrals from social services. Referred children may be those with disabilities, or with other special needs, but are primarily those on the local authority 'at risk' register.

The Save the Children model is grounded in a children's rights perspective on child care policy but remains a minority model among the different types of centre-based family support facilities operated by the voluntary and statutory sector across the country (Hawthorne Kirk 1995). A more in-depth analysis of the different approaches to the development of social welfare services for children and points of convergence between them is provided by Fox Harding (1991).

COMMUNITY ACCESS

The appropriateness of the centres' role can only be judged in the light of the centres' success in making contact with those sections of the community they aim to reach. Save the Children's commitment to equal opportunities entails that community access takes account of child and adult users' and potential users' racial background and ethnic and religious affiliation, their gender and sexual orientation, and differing abilities.

The issues surrounding community access to these centres were analysed by Statham (1994) in terms of who is able to use them, who is allowed to, and who wants to use them. The 1993 review confirmed that staffing ratios and space limitations imposed practical constraints on community access, with waiting lists operating for most of the early-years services and priority being given to certain categories of users, including referrals from social services or health visitors.

Services catered primarily for young children and women, while young people had special facilities provided for them in only about half of the centres. The difficulty in providing opportunities for adolescents was generally deplored by managers. A few projects identified needs among gay and lesbian parents in their area, which were being met to some extent.

Project managers were aware of groups within the community who did not feel comfortable using the centres, such as adult men or certain ethnic groups. Overall, managers felt that their users adequately reflected the ethnic composition of the areas in which the centres were located.

Some centres, like the Hopscotch Asian Women's Centre in the London Borough of Camden, were set up to work with one ethnic group, Bengali women, many of them homeless. But this project was nevertheless concerned that it failed to meet needs, in particular those of other Bengali groups within this community, such as older women and young men.

Centres were also aware of groups they were failing to reach, such as Travellers, and the need to devise strategies to draw such groups into the centres' orbit. In the case of Travellers, Save the Children has a history of operating a variety of non-centre-based family support services for them, or has been working with the Traveller community from bases smaller than the centres that were reviewed.

Management was united in the view that access for children and adults with disabilities was unsatisfactory, although the majority of centres integrated children and young people with disabilities into centre services or provided advice to them. However, even those centres catering for these groups regarded services as insufficient and felt that these groups were not yet properly represented among users.

Architectural features hampered access for users with mobility problems to some centres, while in others it appeared that more outreach work was needed to alert families to the opportunities on offer for children and young people with disabilities. The Strabane family centre in Northern Ireland not only offered disabled access, but also provided transport to bring in users from across a wide area.

Since the review was conducted, practice guidelines on disability have been adopted in the UK, which go some way to countering these problems, while some centres were adapted or moved to new premises.

The disability access problem is not unique to Save the Children centres. The Audit Commission (1994: 26) noted that in the centres they visited, children with disabilities 'were not present unless disabilities appeared specifically among the criteria for admission', even in centres which were both equipped and willing to integrate them.

None of the centres catered for families living in a rural area, so this aspect of equal opportunities in access did not get adequately explored in the review. Rural child care needs, though, were the subject of an earlier Save the Children research initiative (Esslemont and Harrison 1991) in Wales.

Empowerment of the community lies at the root of anti-racist and other anti-discriminatory practice as found in Save the Children centres, but will not be explored further in this chapter. However, this concept in community development is discussed extensively by Warren in Chapter 5.

FAMILY SUPPORT AND THE NOTION OF PREVENTION

Centre-based family support has been explicitly recognised in the Children Act as a service to be encouraged and supported by local authorities, not only in relation to children 'in need', but also to 'a wide range of families' and 'children of all ages' (Smith 1992: 9). This recognition of family centres as a necessary and important component of a children's services system is of crucial importance in the sustainability of Save the Children centres.

Cannan is among those who acknowledge that, while family support centres should form part of a universalist service, there should actually be room in them for families referred for problems of a more personal nature such as serious parenting problems. That this may not be easy because of tensions between different types of users, is brought out in studies by Stones (1989, 1994) and Gill (1988). They looked at a multi-purpose family centre run by Barnardo's, to examine the effect on parents and children of providing a mixture of therapeutic and more general social support. Similar observations were made by Ferri and Saunders (1993) who studied some other Barnardo's centres.

There is support from research for the effectiveness of the approach to prevention adopted by Save the Children. Comparing the needs of families using six family centres operated by The Children's Society, Smith (1993) found the differences between 'open access' for families using the centres in her study and those referred to them to be much less than expected, while all had considerable needs, in particular the one-parent families among them.

This finding was in line with earlier research based on the National Child Development Study by Wedge (1983), research on preventive social work in practice by Gardner (1992) and studies by Tunstill (1992). This led Smith to conclude that

> no preventive strategy can limit itself to reacting to those at any particular time already 'in the net', so to speak, but must be more broadly proactive with respect to those likely to be at risk at some time in the future.

(Smith 1993: 18)

Gibbons (1990) reviewed the literature on the aims and effectiveness of family support pre-dating the implementation of the Children Act. She found that outcome studies of family support programmes were mostly inconclusive. But the scarcity of controlled evaluations of the effectiveness of measures aimed at preventing serious childrearing problems and the removal of children from home was particularly striking.

Holman (1992) acknowledges that open-access centres operate with a different kind of preventive agenda from the more narrowly focused ones aimed only at children 'at risk', but with potentially equal impact. Gibbons argued for measuring the effectiveness of such centres using different and relevant criteria such as 'their contribution to decreasing social isolation among families and increasing social integration' (Gibbons 1990: 32). Social isolation has been identified widely in research, according to Hearn, as a factor which 'often underpins the deterioration into physical abuse and neglect' (Hearn 1995: 19).

An indirect case for the likelihood of such centres reaching the intended population at least as well as targeted services was made by Little and Gibbons (1993). They demonstrated that the outcomes of traditional approaches to child protection meant that, in England and Wales, only a small proportion of ill-treated children were registered as at risk, as a result of the adoption of different registration criteria and the different styles of investigation by different levels of staff.

Even the Audit Commission sanctioned a broad-based approach to the delivery of community-based family support, concluding that family centres could provide a 'one stop shop' for local communities if based in appropriate locations (1994: 39). However, it did not pay specific attention to the role of sessional and full day care in such facilities, although several of the facilities examined did in fact offer this.

Yet, of all the different services forming part of such a preventative family support package, the case for day care as an essential component has been most strongly supported by research. But the short- and long-term effectiveness of the provision of day care in improving the quality of life for young children and their families, has not been widely researched (Macdonald and Roberts 1995).

DAY CARE AS PART OF CENTRE-BASED FAMILY SUPPORT

Day care, both sessional in crèches and playgroup sessions, as well as full-time in day-nursery facilities, has been the cornerstone of centre-based family support provided by Save the Children. Its effect on young children's development, their quality of life as well as on their parents' skills and well-being was evaluated by Thomas (1995) in the Cynon Valley project in Wales.

This project, offering sessional day care for children from the age of 30 months and drop-ins for parents with children under 3 was studied by Thomas over the first five years of its existence. It is used by residents of two deprived estates high up the valley in one of the former mining areas of Mid Glamorgan. The project was shown to help reduce isolation for parents and children and to offer them an opportunity to meet other families and support each other.

How important this is to parents in helping them cope better with the demands of parenting also emerged from Smith's (1993) study of six family centres. The parents interviewed by Smith overwhelmingly wanted the centres to provide play opportunities and day care as well as the chance for them to meet with other parents for support and socialisation. Parents regretted the fact that day care was offered in few of these centres.

In Gibbons's study of the effectiveness of two different styles of delivering social services in two neighbourhoods, 'The evidence suggested that the support of family, friends and neighbours, and the use of day care provision, might have been as or more important in reducing personal stress caused by high levels of family problems' (Gibbons 1990: 149) than other interventions on offer.

Gibbons (1991) also researched the outcome of referrals to social services over a four month period. She found that the provision of day care was the only intervention with a significant positive effect on outcomes for both parents and children, in particular for lone parents.

Finally, in devising their day care programmes for children, Save the

Children operates on the premise that 'for young children, care and education are interdependent and inseparable: they need both' (Sylva and Moss 1992: 1). Projects try to ensure that provision meets the curriculum quality criteria now being set for early-years services, including integrated care and education facilities for young children, with a special emphasis on equal opportunities practice.

THE ROLE OF THE CENTRE IN FAMILY SUPPORT

Regardless of the accumulating evidence for the effectiveness of centre-based family support, there are economic, practical and ideological reasons which may lead policy makers and practitioners to question the necessity of delivering family support from a centre base. Can such support not be delivered equally effectively from a number of different, smaller and more specialised bases within communities? Or from one small base?

Strong arguments are available to support the position that the sum of centre-based family support services is greater than its parts, that the centre lends strength and acts as a resource to other family support activities in the community and that its impact derives to a large extent from this particular method of delivery.

The different forms of outreach work undertaken from Save the Children centres depend on services and facilities provided at 'base' to sustain them. Also, families contacted in the community are put in touch in this way with people and provisions at the centre. However, the size of the base may vary in relation to a particular community's needs.

For instance, the Langley Children's project, a partnership initiative on the boundary between Rochdale and Manchester, operates from a relatively small centre base, and a number of even smaller bases around the community, providing sessional day care and out-of-school services.

In the case of 'satellite' services like the support for child minders in the community provided by Trinity House in Manchester, the project team and its users can again tap into resources that would not normally be available if the child-minding support scheme within the project were completely independent in terms of location and management. A focus on community-health needs at the Cowgate Children's Centre in Newcastle and the Pennywell Neighbourhood Centre in Sunderland, means that difficult to reach services find a firm base within the community they serve.

Carr (1995) contrasted a non-centre-based community development approach to family support provision run by one worker, with a centre-based 'therapeutic' family centre in Newcastle. Although both projects were supported by Save the Children, neither took part in the 1993 review, due to a local management decision. Carr concluded that

> The ideal family support provision would probably exhibit aspects of both projects: a base and trained staff to deal with particular families, offering a wide programme and access to other services, with an outreach element which attempted to develop community development approaches to meeting those general needs experienced by local families.
>
> (Carr 1995: 29)

As far as the needs and wishes of users themselves are concerned, one centre catering for children of different ages as well as for adults can be preferable to different services for different age groups located in various places, especially for families with very young children, for obvious logistical reasons.

Scott (1989), referred to in Pugh (1992), noted that when Scottish parents had been given the option of new and extended early-years provision, they had expressed a preference for multi-functional centres combining early education and day care. While in another Scottish study, parents thought that 'family support should be an integral part of all early years services' (Hawthorne Kirk 1995: 115).

There would appear to be economies of scale in providing services from one centre base, using a centre and community-network model, and indeed it may otherwise be impossible to sustain the full range of outreach, satellite and centre-based services on offer. In practice, such a centre could also itself be attached to a school (Pugh and McQuail 1995), or it could cater for wider needs in the community, such as those of the elderly population (Cannan 1992).

However, experience and policy analysis combined demonstrate that scaling up from existing provision will prove impossible in the absence of a secure funding base grounded in a national early-childhood policy and strategy (Statham 1994; Pugh and McQuail 1995). That such a system could have clear pay-offs for the economy has been demonstrated by Cohen and Fraser (1991), Schweiwe (1994) and Holtermann (1995a).

MULTI-FUNCTIONAL CENTRES IN EUROPE

In a European context, Moss (1992) described the diversification of existing but separate services into multi-functional services as the way forward, if the needs of a broader range of children and their carers were to be met. In practice, this would mean extending day nurseries or family centres

> to become multi-functional centres in their area. This approach breaks down not only the care education divide, but the tendency to fragment services, conceptually and in practice.

> (Moss 1992: 43)

In Europe, the trend towards targeting of this particular type of children's service has been successfully resisted so far, and they form part of a wider children's services system. In Denmark and Sweden (Hwang 1991), a choice of both multi-functional child care centres and separate pre- and out-of-school centres meet community demand, including that for places for children 'in need'. The former type of provision outnumbers the latter, however.

The viability of financial and practical partnerships with the private sector in such ventures elsewhere in Europe has also been demonstrated, particularly where they are based in the community and underpinned by public funding (Cohen 1993). Yet even there reductions in public funding are having an effect, particularly on services for the very youngest children (Combe 1992).

Do rural child care needs contradict the usefulness of the centre-based model of delivering family support? Research in Scotland (Palmer 1991) concluded that evidence from Scottish as well as Danish and French rural provision confirmed that multi-functional centres could even here provide the most promising policy option for the future. Palmer observed that the flexibility offered by age-integrated centres made them more likely to be financially viable in rural areas.

The Save the Children type of multi-functional and multi-professional centre can be said to reflect a European model, where it is seen as an essential component of a system of early-childhood services. Such centres may embrace a wide range of services and facilities, including some for sections of the community other than families with young children.

As far as Save the Children's centres are concerned, the flexibility that allows the centres to interpret the broad principles on which they operate

> to suit their local situation, seems to be a key factor in making them responsive to local need. Just as there is no one model of a disadvantaged area, there is unlikely to be one way of providing services that is appropriate in all situations.

> (Statham 1994: 38)

Recent policy research confirms that Save the Children's approach to centre-based family support does address all factors identified as important in planning and delivering such services. For instance, in their study of the co-ordination of children's services in eleven local authorities with different organisational structures, Pugh and McQuail (1995) conclude that the boundaries between day care services, child protection and family support must be bridged, irrespective of the model adopted.

The Save the Children centres do all these things and thereby lead the way in the trend towards multi-functional centres of the kind noted in continental Europe.

FACING THE FUTURE

Secure long-term funding would be needed for planing around existing voluntary, statutory and private provision and stimulating the development of new forms that would generate an effectively organised system of complementary and integrated child care services for communities. It therefore ultimately depends on a national child care policy and strategic planning on the part of local and central government (Ball 1994; Holtermann 1995b; Pugh and McQuail 1995).

The Save the Children centres try and reconcile ways of delivering family support that can only be truly effective if delivered within a system of universal early-years services based on sustained public funding. Its centre-based family support finds itself in the same position as local authority provision in Scotland described by Hawthorne Kirk:

> The continuing absence of central government funding, direction and mandate to provide pre-school services, allows the conflicting perspectives embodied by local authority services to be perpetuated, i.e. rationing and targeting on the one hand and universalism and equal opportunities on the other. Many of them are in an impossible position, trying as they do, to satisfy the challenges made from both directions.
> (Hawthorne Kirk 1995: 115)

She argues that an even more comprehensive approach is needed to address the multiple types of deprivation communities suffer, as do Cannan (1992), and Deccio et al. (1994). Statutory and non-statutory agencies should not only encourage participation in community groups and activities, but also create employment opportunities for adults in low-income families.

In their provision of educational, training and employment opportunities, such as in the Rosemount and Patmore centres in Glasgow and

London (Laws 1995), Save the Children centres have taken one important step further in a direction identified by these authors as going beyond the interpersonal dimension of social support, and addressing structural elements such as poverty and unemployment. However, it would seem that by doing so, centre-based family support in Save the Children has made itself even more vulnerable to the vagaries of politics, funding policies and the economic climate.

The different strands of evidence produced in this chapter support the case for the effectiveness and appropriateness of Save the Children's model of centre-based family support, although it is acknowledged that there is a need for research into its longer term outcomes for children and their families.

A number of urgent challenges present themselves to its sustainability. The onus is now on central and local government to work together with the voluntary and private sectors in securing the future of what is increasingly being seen as an essential component in a system of services responsive to the needs of young children and their families.

REFERENCES

Audit Commission (1994) *Seen but not Heard: Co-ordinating Community Child Health and Social Services for Children in Need, Detailed Evidence and Guidelines for Managers and Practitioners*, London: HMSO.
Ball, C. (1994) *Start Right: The Importance of Early Learning*, London: Royal Society of Arts.
Barclay, P. (1995) *Joseph Rowntree Foundation Inquiry into Income and Wealth*, York: Joseph Rowntree Foundation.
Bradshaw, J. (1992) *Child Poverty and Deprivation in the UK*, London: National Children's Bureau for UNICEF.
Cannan, C. (1992) *Changing Families, Changing Welfare: Family Centres and the Welfare State*, New York/London: Harvester Wheatsheaf.
Carr, J. (1995) *Family Support: Two Approaches – Centre and Community*, Leeds: Save the Children.
Cohen, B. (1993) *Childcare in Partnership: Local Authority/Employer Partnership Initiatives in the European Community*, Brussels: Commission of the European Communities.
Cohen, B. and Fraser, N. (1991) *Childcare in a Modern Welfare System*, London: Institute for Public Policy Research.
Combe, J. (1992) *Parent Run Day Care Centres: the Growth of a French Community Initiative*, The Hague: Bernard van Leer Foundation Studies and Evaluation Papers 8.
De'Ath, E. (1988) *Focus on Families: The Family Centre Approach*, Children's Society Briefing Paper, London: The Children's Society.
Deccio, G., Horner, W. C. and Wilson, D. (1994) 'High-risk neighbourhoods and high-risk families: replication research related to the human ecology of child maltreatment', *Journal of Social Services Research*, 18 (3/4): 123–37

Department of Health (1991) *The Children Act 1989 Guidance and Regulations: Vol. 2, Family Support, Day Care and Educational Provision for Young Children*, London: HMSO.

Earls, F., McGuire, J. and Shay, S. (1994) 'Evaluating a community intervention to reduce the risk of child abuse: methodological strategies in conducting neighbourhood surveys', *Child Abuse and Neglect*, 18 (5): 473–85.

Esslemont, E. and Harrison, J. (1991) *Swings and Roundabouts: the Highs and Lows of Life for Pre-School Children and their Families in Rural Powys*, Cardiff: Save the Children/ Cronfa Achub y Plant.

Ferri, E. and Niblett, R. (1977) *Disadvantaged Families and Playgroups*, An NCB Report, Windsor: NFER Nelson Publishing Company.

Ferri, E. and Saunders, A. (1993) *Parents, Professionals and Pre-school Centres: A Study of Barnardo's Provision*, London: National Children's Bureau and Barnardo's.

Finch, J. (1983) 'Can skills be shared? Pre-school playgroups in disadvantaged areas', *Community Development Journal*, 18 (3): 251–6.

Fox Harding, E. (1991) *Perspectives on Childcare*, London: Longman.

Garbarino, J. and Kostelny, K. (1992) 'Child maltreatment as a community problem', *Child Abuse and Neglect*, 16: 455–64.

Gardner, R. (1992) *Supporting Families: Preventive Social Work in Action*, London: National Children's Bureau.

Gibbons, J. with Thorpe, S. and Wilkinson, P. (1990) *Family Support and Prevention: Studies in Local Areas*, London: HMSO.

Gibbons, J. (1991) 'Children in need and their families: outcomes of referral to social services', *British Journal of Social Work*, 21: 217–27.

Gibbons, J. (ed.) (1992) *The Children Act 1989 and Family Support: Principles into Practice*, London: HMSO.

Gill, O. (1988) 'Integrated work in a neighbourhood family centre', *Practice*, 2 (3): 243–55.

Hardiker, P., Exton, K. and Barker, M. (1995) *The Prevention of Child Abuse: A Framework for Analysing Services*, London: The National Commission of Inquiry into the Prevention of Child Abuse.

Hawthorne Kirk, R. (1995) 'Social support and early years centres', in M. Hill, R. Hawthorne Kirk and D. Part (eds), *Supporting Families*, Edinburgh: HMSO.

Hearn, B. (1995) *Child and Family Support and Protection: A Practical Approach*, London: National Children's Bureau.

Holman, B. (1988) *Putting Families First: Prevention and Child Care*, London: Macmillan Educational.

Holman, B. (1992) 'Linking up with the locals', *Community Care*, July: 14–15.

Holtermann, S. (1995a) *Investing in Young Children: A Reassessment of the Cost of an Education and Day Care Service*, London: National Children's Bureau, on behalf of the Statutory and Voluntary Young Children Group.

Holtermann, S. (1995b) *All our Futures: The Impact of Public Expenditure and Fiscal Policies on Britain's Children and Young People*, Barkingside: Barnardo's.

Hwang, P. (1991) 'Day care in Sweden', in P. Moss and E. Melhuish (eds), *Current Issues in Day Care for Young Children*, London: HMSO.

Jackson, C. (1986) *Family Centres Survey*, London: Save the Children Fund, on behalf of the National Council for Voluntary Child Care Organisations.

Jones, A. and Bilton, K. (1994) *Shape Up or Shake Up: The Future of Services for Children in Need*, London: National Children's Bureau.

Joseph, A. and Parfitt, J. (1972) *Playgroups in an Area of Social Need*, An NCB Report, Windsor: NFER Nelson Publishing Company.

Kumar, V. (1993) *Poverty and Inequality in the UK: The Effects on Children*, London: National Children's Bureau.

Laws, S. (1995) *Lasting Benefits for Children: Education and Training for Women*, London: Save the Children.

Little, M. and Gibbons, J. (1993) 'Predicting the rate of children on the child protection register', *Research, Policy and Planning*, 10 (2): 15–18.

Lloyd, E. (1993) *Save the Children Centres: Families, Children, Resource, the 1993 Review, a Paper for Discussion*, London: Save the Children.

Lloyd, E., Melhuish, E., Moss, P. and Owen, C. (1989) 'A review of research on playgroups', *Early Child Development and Care*, 43: 77–99.

Long, G. (1995) 'Family poverty and the role of family support work', in M. Hill, R. Hawthorne Kirk and D. Part (eds), *Supporting Families*, Edinburgh: HMSO.

Macdonald, G. and Roberts, H. (1995) *What Works in the Early Years: Effective Interventions For Children and Families in Health, Social Welfare, Education and Child Protection*, Barkingside: Barnardo's.

Moss, P. (1992) 'Perspectives from Europe', in G. Pugh (ed.), *Contemporary Issues in the Early Years*, London: Paul Chapman Publishing.

Oppenheim, C. (1994) *Poverty, the Facts*, London: Child Poverty Action Group.

Palmer, J. (1991) *Childcare in Rural Communities*, Edinburgh: Scottish Child and Family Alliance.

Pugh, G. (ed.) (1992) *Contemporary Issues in the Early Years*, London: Paul Chapman Publishing.

Pugh, G. and McQuail, S. (1995) *Effective Organisation of Early Childhood Services: Summary and Strategic Framework*, London: National Children's Bureau.

Schweiwe, K. (1994) 'Labour market, welfare state and family institutions: the links to mothers' poverty risks; a comparison between Belgium, Germany and the United Kingdom', *Journal of European Social Policy*, 4 (3): 201–24.

Scott, G. (1989) *Families and Under Fives in Strathclyde*, Glasgow: Glasgow College and Strathclyde Regional Council.

Smith, T. (1992) 'Family centres, children in need and the Children Act 1989', in J. Gibbons (ed.) *The Children Act 1989 and Family Support: Principles into Practice*, London: HMSO.

Smith, T. (1993) *Family Centres and Bringing up Young Children: Six Projects Run by the Children's Society*, London: Children's Society and Department of Health.

Smith, T. and Noble, M. (1995) *Education Divides: Poverty and Schooling in the 1990s*, London: Child Poverty Action Group.

Statham, J. (1994) *Childcare in the Community: The Provision of Community Based, Open Access Services for Young Children in Family Centres*, London: Save the Children.

Stones, C. (1989) 'Groups and groupings in a family centre', in A. Brown and R. Clough (eds), *Groups and Groupings: Life and Work in Day and Residential Centres*, London: Tavistock/Routledge.

Stones, C. (1994) *Family Centres in Action*, London: Macmillan.

Sylva, K. and Moss, P. (1992) *Learning before School*, London: National Commission on Education Briefing No 8.

Thomas, A. (1995) *But What About the Children?* Cardiff: Save the Children/ Cronfa Achub y Plant.

Tunstill, J. (1992) 'Local authority policies on children in need', in J. Gibbons (ed.), *The Children Act 1989 and Family Support: Principles into Practice*, London: HMSO.

Walker, H. (1991) 'Family centres', in P. Carter, T. Jeffs and M. Smith (eds), *Social Work and Social Welfare Yearbook 3*, Milton Keynes: Open University Press.

Warren, C. (1991) 'Family centres', in Family Rights Group (ed.), *The Children Act 1989, Working in Partnership with Families: A Reader*, London: HMSO.

Warren, C. (1993) *Family Centres and the Children Act 1989: A Training and Development Handbook*, Arundel: Tarrant Publishing Ltd.

Wedge, P. (1983) 'Some structural factors in social disadvantage: findings from a longitudinal study of children', in M. Brown (ed.), *The Structure of Disadvantage*, SSRC/DHSS Studies in Deprivation and Disadvantage, London: Heinemann.

Williams, P. (1993) *Long-term Funding for Community Projects*, London: Save the Children.

Chapter 8

Mechanisms for empowerment

Family group conferences and local family advocacy schemes

Jo Tunnard

INTRODUCTION

The Children Act 1989 challenged local authorities to identify and provide for the needs of children and their families, rather than focus on parental shortcomings. It requires a redirection away from targeted services for children at risk of abuse, towards universal provision of services aimed at reducing stress on families and the need for crisis intervention. It demands that children and their families play a greater part in planning for their future, and that services reflect the lessons learnt from consulting with the community about their needs.

For families, empowerment is best seen as both a process and a goal. Changed practice in the wake of the 1989 Act should be characterised by people having the power to express their needs and deciding how those needs can best be met.

Some local authorities and voluntary agencies are making progress on both counts. This chapter describes two mechanisms for empowerment that have been developed under the auspices of the Family Rights Group (FRG), a national organisation with a long-standing reputation for promoting user participation in children and family services.

The first is the family group conference (FGC), an exciting concept introduced recently from New Zealand. The chapter describes its development and philosophy, its introduction to the UK, the results emerging from research studies, and how it works in practice.

The second model for empowerment is family advocacy. Family advocacy schemes provide a means of redressing the imbalance of power between statutory agencies and service users. The second part of the chapter describes the slow growth of advocacy in children and family work, the impetus provided by the new legislation, some examples of local work, and the essential elements for successful family advocacy schemes.

This chapter is a collective effort, for it brings together extracts from FRG's recent writings on both family group conferences and family advocacy schemes. Special thanks are due to those whose work is included here – Kate Morris, FRG's lead worker on FGCs; Alison Richards, FRG's lead worker on family advocacy; Murray Ryburn, Senior Lecturer in the Department of Social Work at the University of Birmingham; and Glyn Hughes, Principal Officer, Gwynedd Social Services Department.

FAMILY GROUP CONFERENCES

The family group conference draws kinship groups together in a formal way to entrust them, rather than groups of professionals, with the task of ensuring the safety and welfare of their children. There is nothing novel in the idea of kinship groups meeting to make decisions for their children. What is new is its formalisation as a way of working in situations where social workers and other professionals have been accustomed to the belief that responsibility for making decisions necessarily lies with them.

FGCs originated in New Zealand and were developed initially as a means of meeting the needs of Maori children and families. Their success led to their inclusion in primary legislation (the Children, Young Persons and their Families Act 1989) and to their use for all families, and in all areas of children and family work, including care, protection, and youth justice.

Developing FGCs in the UK

The model is being piloted at present in the UK. This came about as a result of a group of New Zealand practitioners being invited here in 1990 to talk about family group conferences. In view of the enormous potential the model offered for increasing partnership work between professionals and families, FRG undertook to promote the use of FGCs in the UK, securing funding in 1992 to develop this work over a three-year period.

The starting point was the setting up of a national pilot project group convened and supported by FRG. The group consists of seven representatives of local authorities and voluntary agencies. In these areas and agencies workers have run local schemes of FGCs and, through bi-monthly meetings, group members have shared their experiences and developed a body of knowledge and expertise.

One development from the pilot group has been the establishment of a national research group. This group includes those involved in evaluating the local projects as well as others with a general interest in researching the model. The group has aimed to collect compatible data, and recent funding by the Nuffield Foundation has provided a senior researcher, based at Sheffield University under the guidance of Peter Marsh, to support and advise the group.

A third national group is focused on the use of FGCs in youth justice work. Convened by FRG and the National Association for the Care and Rehabilitation of Offenders (NACRO), this group is still in its infancy. It aims to encourage and support the piloting of FGCs in work with young offenders.

The level of professional and public interest in family group conferences is growing. Those involved so far in developing the model in the UK remain excited about the potential they offer to most children and their families for creating plans in partnership with professionals.

The model, while retaining the key features of the New Zealand system, has been adapted to reflect UK law and practice. In addition, the 'home-grown' model lends itself well to being modified to reflect local needs.

There are, however, three crucial elements that must be present for the term 'family group conference' to be appropriate. These are:

- that the term 'family' is interpreted widely, and includes relatives, friends, and other significant people;
- that the family always has the opportunity to plan in private; and
- that the family's plan is agreed by the professionals unless, and only unless, the plan places the child at risk of significant harm.

The mechanics of FGCs

There are four stages to an FGC.

- *The preliminary stage* is the referral of the case to an independent co-ordinator who convenes the FGC. Independent means that the person has no case work or management involvement in the matter. The family is identified, in consultation with the child and their immediate carers, and the meeting is held at a time and venue chosen by the family. The co-ordinator has the right to exclude family members and, where needed, advocates can be identified for vulnerable family members.
- *Stage one* is the start of the FGC meeting. The professionals involved tell the family about the concerns they have for the child, the information that gives rise to those concerns, and the duties and

responsibilities that govern their work. The co-ordinator chairs this part of the meeting and, as throughout the process, the language used is the first language of the family. The onus is on the professionals to use interpreters if they need to. The professionals and the co-ordinator then leave the meeting.

- *Stage two* is time for the family to plan in private. Their task is to agree a plan for their child's care and protection. They are also asked to devise ways of reviewing their plan and to consider contingency plans in case things do not work out as expected.

- *Stage three* starts when the family have agreed their plan and the professionals rejoin the meeting. The plan is agreed and any resources negotiated. The only ground for rejecting the plan is that the plan places the child at risk of significant harm. Should this be the case, either the family reconsiders their plan or the case is referred on to child protection procedures or court proceedings.

The philosophy behind FGCs

When New Zealand implemented its Children, Young Persons and their Families Act in November 1989, it introduced a model for decision making in child care and protection that was unique in Western jurisdictions. This is not to say that each key element of the legislation is necessarily novel, indeed many find echoes in our own Children Act. What is novel, however, is the obligatory role the New Zealand legislation creates for kinship decision making in all instances where young people are deemed to be in need of care and protection. The legislation has a baseline assumption that if families are given the right resources and sufficient knowledge of the facts and the concerns of the professionals, they can make good and wise decisions for their children.

In many respects the New Zealand Act shares a common philosophy with our Children Act, but in its approach to actual practice its uniqueness becomes apparent. Unlike the Children Act, it is prescriptive in establishing a single and unified model for dealing with circumstances where children and young people are thought to be at risk. In doing so it gives a fundamentally clearer and more important role to family groups in making their own decisions about care and protection and, as a result, the professional role is correspondingly redefined and circumscribed.

The prescriptiveness of the New Zealand Act creates a difference that makes a difference. In practice, it means that the spirit of partnership *implicit* in the Children Act is significantly more *explicit* in the New Zealand legislation. Professionals in New Zealand, like their counterparts in England and Wales, have to operate within a new legal framework. In contrast, however, it is not a framework which can be bolted relatively readily on to existing values, attitudes and beliefs. In comparison with mainstream permanence philosophy, where professional expertise and the professional decision-making role are afforded primacy, the New Zealand Act has mandated a new approach for professionals in their dealings with families. The professional role has become much more that of skilled facilitator and resource provider. The greatest importance of this change is that although initially it may not bring about attitudinal changes, over time it may well do so.

The New Zealand legislation is unique in its consistent and explicit acknowledgement of the importance for each child of a family network that is wider than immediate kin, and in recognising throughout that the services and the provisions of the Act must be written and interpreted in ways that are relevant to a multi-cultural community.

Under the New Zealand legislation, no social worker can be left with any doubt that children's own wider kin groups are always the preferred and primary placement option, and that there is something distinctive and special about children's own families that must be preserved. The legislation requires of professionals a new approach, and it puts families at the forefront of planning and decision making in a way that the Children Act just as significantly fails to do. The model is a reassertion of traditional social work skills of facilitation, mediation and enablement. As such, it lies close to social work's cardinal value of respect for persons (Plant 1970).

The shift that it has accomplished on the part of professionals is perhaps summed up best in a government document for staff about the new process of family decision making:

> A central feature of this new Act is the emphasis it places on the role of kin in making decisions for children. The kinship group is seen as not comprising just the nuclear family, but an extended family group including the child's uncles, aunts and grandparents. The procedures established in the Act are based on the belief that, given the resources, the information, and the power, a family group will make safe and appropriate decisions for children.
>
> The role of professionals such as social workers and doctors should not be to make decisions, but to facilitate decision making, by providing information, resources and expertise which will assist the family group. Professionals will have a crucial role as resource people.
>
> (Department of Social Welfare 1989)

Practice in the UK: a case example

The Parry family (not their real name) have four children. Two children from Mrs Parry's current relationship were living at home with their parents whilst the children of her previous marriage, David (aged 7) and Anna (aged 12), were the subject of care orders following serious physical neglect. They had been living with foster carers for over six years.

Mrs Parry had requested that David and Anna be reunited with her. She had maintained regular contact with them throughout their period in foster care. The local authority had agreed to place the children with the mother and stepfather, under the Placement with Parents Regulations, following the death of the foster mother.

It was at this stage that a referral was made to one of the family group conference co-ordinators. The aim of the FGC was to define the package of services that the family needed to ensure a successful placement home and to establish the basis for the placement agreement.

The conference was attended by both children, and eight family members who included the parents, a grandparent, and aunts and uncles. In addition to the social worker and the team leader, the foster father attended the first part of the meeting and the family decided later that he should also stay during the family deliberations.

During stage one of the FGC a number of key areas which needed to be resolved were outlined for the family. These included:

* the level and nature of future contact between the children and the foster family;
* the support system required to cope with the behavioural difficulties sometimes displayed by Anna;
* the support that David needed, to understand the major changes that had occurred recently in his life;
* the practical support the family would require; and
* some concern about what was seen as poor physical standards of care within the home.

The family addressed these issues and produced a detailed plan which was accepted and resourced by the department. During a later interview about the use of the FGC, Mrs Parry said:

The social worker wanted to know what we needed to cope with looking after the children. We decided we wanted the children to carry on seeing the foster father, so they go to him every Friday afternoon, and the department pays his fares. My mum has them on Saturdays.

They were also worried about David, who is confused about the changes, so my mum and my husband's brother said they would spend time alone with him every week to talk to him about things.

We asked for a lot of practical help. We were living in a flat and asked the department if they could help us get a bigger place from the housing department. In two weeks we were offered a house. We also asked for a washing machine and dryer, and extra bedclothes, and school clothes, as Anna wets her bed every night, and we have got them.

It was good getting the family together to think about the kids. They feel more involved now than they would have been if they had not come to the conference. It is not easy getting used to living together again, but I am so pleased to have them back after all this time, and I think we're managing quite well.

The family also decided to review progress after six months by re-convening the family group conference. Slightly fewer family members attended this meeting, six rather than eight, and, although considerable progress had been made, there were some issues that were causing concern. The family once again addressed these issues and made practical decisions that resolved the concerns. For example, the younger children had been left on their own whilst the mother took the older ones to school. In response, the family established a simple rota to care for the children between eight and nine in the morning.

To date the reunification of the children with their parents has been successful, and progress will continue to be reviewed regularly by the family via the FGC process.

Questions about empowerment in practice

A number of common questions are often raised in relation to FGCs, and two in particular – about children, and about men – pose the question of whether the empowerment of some users leads to a consequent decrease in the power of others.

Are children overlooked?

It is sometimes claimed that the FGC model fails to attach sufficient importance to the paramountcy of children's interests and that these will be submerged if families are allowed to make their own decisions. The idea that the interests of any of us are readily separable from the context of relationships with those who are most important to us is, of course, a nonsense, even when abuse has occurred. It belies the fact that each of us, including children, gives meaning to and interprets best interests only within the framework of those to whom we have significant attachments.

New Zealand practitioners report that children often feel greatly surprised, and find their self-esteem boosted, when they realise that they are sufficiently important for their whole kin network to meet solely to consider their welfare. Children are always invited to FGCs and they can have with them anyone whom they wish to support or speak for them.

The views of professionals about the best interests of children are not lost in the FGC either. They are part of the information that is presented to the first stage of the conference and, in the final stage of the process, it is necessary for the referrer to agree that the family's plan for any child is consistent with the child's welfare. This occurred in 93 per cent of FGCs in the first year of operation in New Zealand (Hassall and Maxwell 1991).

Once professional knowledge and concerns are shared openly with families at the first stage of the conference, the power of the secrets, which usually support abuse or neglect by one or a small number of relatives, is diminished. Families, with their expertise on their own ways of functioning, can then often build protection and safety into care and contact plans in ways that professionals' more limited knowledge of the family and its dynamics may prevent their achieving.

Does male power get reinforced?

Critics of the model have sometimes argued that it replaces paternalism (the state deciding) with patriarchy, since in many families in different cultures men exercise decision making power over women and children. An added criticism is that it is the exercise of this power by men that is at the heart of much abuse, particularly sexual abuse.

It is undoubtedly true that the family, as socially constructed in many different cultures, serves to reinforce the dominance of male interests. Unfortunately, the same is true of other social structures and organisations. Social work is a profession served largely by women but managed predominantly by men, and so the same critique can be made of professional social work decisions about what is best for children. This point is made, not to minimise the criticism of the FGC but, rather, to highlight the importance of finding new ways of redressing the imbalances that dominate so much of our work.

The FGC model can present a more effective challenge to the male domination that leads to the abuse of women and children. The public disclosure of abuse, to members of the wider family, helps to destroy the tacit acceptance of male power that can be necessary for its perpetuation. Experience of the FGC model has shown that it can create opportunities for women, across generations, to establish new coalitions in order to protect children. The support and sanction of these plans by professionals can contribute to women gaining greater power in situations where men have been abusers.

Some early research findings

UK research in child care practice has shown that when professionals remain in charge of the decision-making process, all too often they fail to consult adequately and they make decisions, whether planned or as a consequence of professional inactivity, that then fail children and their families (see, for example, Fruin and Vernon 1986; Millham *et al.* 1986, 1989; Fisher *et al.* 1986; Berridge and Cleaver 1987).

Findings so far from the FGC pilot project suggest a number of key practice points.

- Venue is important. Preferably it should be neutral, and comfortable. Families stress the provision of adequate facilities as important in making their meeting feel credible and valued.
- Preparation is crucial. If done well, all stages of the FGC will go much more smoothly.
- It is important to give time to the last stage of the FGC, when the family reports back about their plan. If this is rushed, and details not discussed, plans may not be so effective.
- Families need to be told that they can go on to request further FGCs. It is also important to call a re-convened meeting a 'family group conference' so families do not feel that the meeting has been down-graded.
- Some family members report the process to be very difficult, but are equally clear that it was helpful and much preferred to other, existing, decision-making processes such as child protection conferences.
- Family plans do not necessarily differ greatly from professionals' plans. What may differ is who implements the plan. Families might choose to use other family members in roles, such as befrienders and respite carers, that historically would have been undertaken by non-family members.
- FGCs are not a 'cheap option'. The aim is not to cut costs by using family resources. The family plan should be negotiated and resourced appropriately. Families might identify and use resources that profes-

sionals had not considered, such as placements within the child's network. These plans will still need resourcing, and that will include practical and financial assistance.

- FGCs are about the *way* in which plans are made. The plans produced will vary in style, content and cost, according to the particular needs of the child. Plans should reflect issues such as race, culture and religion, and move us away from professional-dominated outcomes.
- The role of the co-ordinator is crucial in achieving an effective process and outcome.

The role of the co-ordinator

We end with the views of one co-ordinator about what he has learnt so far in using this exciting new way of empowering families.

The importance of stressing the independence of the co-ordinator. . . . I feel it was useful that I am not employed by a statutory authority, and had no other responsibility with the situation but to enable and empower the family to meet and make decisions.

The importance of perseverance. Some of the extended family needed three or four visits by appointment to see someone about the conference. Family members are busy, and have very different priorities – an extended work shift or a problem with a neighbour can seem more important than meeting someone they don't know to discuss an extended family member who is perceived as a problem.

The realisation that from the moment you start the process, something is happening in the family that would not otherwise have happened. People are contacting each other about your visit; some family members are beginning to feel involved for the first time in years; some people are feeling threatened and challenged by the invitation to participate. There is a process that begins with the very first contact, not just the content outcome of the conference.

The importance of the belief in the family and its ability to take power for itself and produce a plan that is at least as good, and probably more creative and potentially effective, than that produced by the 'professionals'.

The crucial role played by the advocate of the child. The child's choice in this is important. I was amazed at the competence and effectiveness of using another young person to help her friend speak and be heard in a group of vocal adults.

The tremendous buzz that is felt by the family, and infects the professionals, when a family believes in itself and produces a plan to present to social services.

The importance of the support and training group for co-ordinators. It would be difficult to work in isolation, without the opportunity to share experiences and consolidate learning that this offers.

FAMILY ADVOCACY SCHEMES

Advocacy projects have been in existence around health and welfare issues for well over a decade in Britain and, more recently, they have been extended to groups and individuals with physical disabilities and learning difficulties. So, there are schemes that:

* provide parents with an advocacy service for their children with learning, hearing, mobility or language difficulties;
* offer a befriending and representation service for people who have suffered mental health problems;
* represent the users of psychiatric services on issues of concern about treatment; and
* offer advocacy about welfare benefits. Local welfare benefit units have made great progress in providing information, representing individuals and client groups, influencing the take-up of benefits, challenging decisions at local tribunals and the High Court and European Court, and acting as a consumer watchdog on central government legislation and local interpretation.

The gap for families

Despite the prominent part played by such schemes in the provision of health and social services, advocacy has been poorly developed as a service to parents and other relatives of children who have been, are, or might become separated from their children through accommodation or care. There have been virtually no locally-based agencies willing or able to provide family members with this specialist information, support and advocacy.

Traditionally, as a result, the best hope of families is that they lived in the catchment area of the few law centres that did care work, or that their social worker or community worker could put them in touch with a solicitor willing to go beyond their normal legal work and accompany family members to planning or appeal meetings. Even then, the tightening of the legal aid criteria disqualifies an increasing number of parents on a low income, or grandparents with even modest savings for their retirement and funeral.

All this has been a cause for great concern, especially when one considers the traumatic impact on people's lives of some of the decisions that can be made by social workers and other professionals. It causes concern, too, because the potential gains for families and their children can be so enormous. Organisations like the Family Rights Group, advocating for children and adults, have often been able to help families gain some improvement in what they believe to be best for their young members. This has included:

- more contact with their child;
- visits in a more relaxed place;
- choice about foster carers and children's homes;
- the chance to attend a meeting about their child's future;
- children placed together with their brothers and sisters;
- written agreements that spell out the work to be done;
- appeal against professional decisions;
- the removal of a child's name from the child protection register;
- the return of a child to parents or other relatives;
- financial help for visits to and from their children;
- interpreters to enable them to understand and participate; and
- getting their voice heard, even though their view might not have prevailed.

Some progress on child advocacy

Advocacy schemes for children in contact with social services began to get established before the Children Act came into force. One early scheme, operating in the London borough of Greenwich, placed emphasis on solving problems before they needed to be dealt with as formal complaints. Children have access to a local youth counselling centre where they can get advice and information and, if necessary, arrangements are made for an independent advocate to be appointed to help them sort out the problem they are having with the social services 'system'. Only if the matter cannot be resolved by discussion, or if the advocacy fails to resolve things satisfactorily, is a formal complaint made.

This scheme was initiated by A Voice for the Child in Care (VCC) and now operates in other parts of England. Important contributions were made also by other organisations such as the National Association for Young People In Care (NAYPIC) and the Children's Legal Centre – both now defunct, the Who Cares? Trust, and Independent Representation for Children in Need (IRCHIN).

These developments mirror practice in the United States where there is a strong tradition of child advocacy, and where much has been written about it. McGowan (1977) has stressed that good advocates need a range of strategies to draw on, that advocacy is a long-term process rather than a speedy answer to problems, and that the most effective advocates are those who focus on specific issues.

Wolfensberger's view (1977) is that all service delivery should include an element of advocacy: those who care for children, the elderly, and others, should all advocate on their behalf with official institutions and agencies. He pioneered the view that advocacy is about speaking on behalf of people with vigour and vehemence, with successful outcomes resulting in power beginning to shift away from professionals, in favour of clients. You know when you are doing it well, he said, because 'whenever advocacy really begins to work it will be persecuted . . . the phonier it is the more likely it is to be praised'.

Local advocacy work for families

Some UK local authorities have used and promoted local support groups as a source of information and advice for families. The common function of these groups is the moral support members offer one another in times of stress – when children are in accommodation or care, or have returned home, or are involved in child protection procedures. But most groups do other things besides. Group members accompany parents to meetings with professional workers. They speak at training sessions for foster carers and social workers, and produce useful guides for families (Parents' Aid 1991).

Some have been consulted on draft policy statements about access, parental contributions and complaints procedures. One had regular meetings for two years with their director of social services. Another helped a couple take their case to the European Court on the grounds that the government had violated their rights to family life because they were denied access to their child and had no legal remedy against that decision. Their success, and that of four other families heard at the same time, helped improve the law on contact between children and their families.

The support groups that provide advocacy services have developed in different ways (Hosie 1985; FRG 1990, 1991). In Newcastle-upon-Tyne the local Families In Care Group employs a part-time worker. The group has long been supported by a local voluntary agency, with the worker funded by the social services department. In Harlow, a local person is employed for a day a week by Parents' Aid, the first self-help group, established in 1979. In Colchester, a local parent runs one session a week in three different places. On Merseyside, the Family Support Association provides advice and advocacy through a full-time and sessional workers. In Norfolk, a group of parents operates with support from the social work department of the local university. In Plymouth, a local support group was one initiative arising from the development work undertaken by the Dartington Social Research Unit in the wake of its research into contact problems for children and their families.

A related development is the growth of the Grandparents' Federation which, on a national basis, offers support and friendship to those whose young relatives are in accommodation or care or have been adopted from care. And a proposal for Neighbourhood Welfare Forums (Holman 1991) added another exciting variation on the theme: officials and politicians would meet in public with service users to discuss policies, practices and, if individuals agree, single cases. To what end? 'Agencies may well improve attitudes to the public if subject to local debate. Just as important, officials and users at last could make common cause for social reforms' (*Guardian*, 12 June 1991).

Self-help groups vary, of course, and they have waxed and waned as family priorities shift. But their existence, and their experiences, are a powerful reminder that being at the receiving end of the state's child care system leaves many of those it affects with an abiding mistrust of people who have authority over others. Too many families know, in ways they carry with them forever, and which outsiders will never fully understand, about the ways people use authority to exclude them from decisions about their children's lives. Few parents have been offered the opportunity to meet other such parents. Yet they have something important and unique to offer one another: a common problem, a sympathetic ear, hope in the face of adversity, consolation when their children are lost to them.

When the University of East Anglia carried out an investigation into parents' aid groups, it pinpointed ways in which social workers and managers can help groups to start and flourish. It recommended the views of local group members to those departments who were looking for ways of improving the effectiveness of their service to families of children in care (Monaco and Thoburn 1987). At a time when research evidence was accumulating about the way families were ignored in the planning for their children's future, and moves were afoot to make more sense of the muddle and mess of children and family legislation, local support groups were seen as having an important contribution to make to the development of user-friendly services based on a philosophy of partnership between professionals and families.

The hopes for advocacy after the Children Act

In its training work on partnership work under the Act, FRG highlighted some of the possible roles of local advocacy schemes:

*   Advocacy could help make a reality of the Act's provisions for user consultation and representation.
*   It could offer an independent source of legal and practice expertise for parents and others, in order to help them become parties to the sort of written agreements that are most likely to work well.
*   It could help ensure that the spirit of partnership continues after compulsory intervention. The support of an advocate would increase the chances of parents retaining their sense of confidence and commitment to the work that is needed once a court order is made, and would thus increase the chances of continuing contact for children and the likelihood of their return home.
*   Advocacy could provide a focal point for information about available services, and about the best source of services for particular families.
*   It could provide a focal point for information about, and access to, self-help groups in the area.
*   It could offer a useful service in relation to local authority charging policies.
*   It lends itself to being a vehicle to strengthen the relationship between individual practice and the organisational structures and systems deriving from the Act. So, local advocates could help press for mechanisms for evaluating services provided. They could lead the way in establishing a framework for recording the unmet needs for family support services under Section 17 of the Act, in recognition of the fact that if all needs cannot be met – irrespective of whether the term is interpreted widely or narrowly – it will be crucial to have a record of what has not been provided, to use in future negotiations around budget allocations. All this was seen as having the potential to enable some social workers, and strengthen others, to see that an essential part of the professional social work task is to make sure that managers, policy makers and elected members are kept well informed about such important issues.

Progress since the Act

It is disappointing to report the slow progress in local authority support for advocacy schemes over the past four years. As before the Act, the most heartening news is about services for children and young people. Several local authorities have appointed children's rights officers whose brief includes information and advocacy to children who are looked after by the local authority; a few have established schemes to respond to the needs of particular groups of looked-after children, such as those in residential care; and a growing number are contracting for the services of specialist advocacy agencies, notably ASC (Advice, Advocacy and Representation Service for Children), based in Manchester and providing a telephone help-line and individual advocates, predominantly for young people in residential and foster placements.

But for adult family members, there is still next to nothing on offer. A trawl of UK social work departments confirmed our fears that no area is providing current and potential service users with adequate access to specialist advocacy services. It is to be hoped that FRG's current family advocacy project (FRG 1995) – funded by the BBC Children In Need Appeal, and designed to help six areas develop local schemes – will provide the much-needed impetus for this work. Work is in progress with a mixture of local authority and voluntary sector projects in Wiltshire, Wigan, Norwich, Oxford, Newham and Walthamstow.

A local example: planning for family advocacy in Hackney

During 1995 FRG has been offering Hackney Social Services Department (SSD) a specialist consultancy, working alongside one of their four area family support managers, helping the borough establish an advocacy service for current and potential users of its children and family service. Most of the work has been done with the help and support of an active and committed steering group. This was set up at the start of the project, and consists of workers in voluntary organisations, local health and disability advocates, social services specialist workers, a local solicitor and service users.

The following paragraphs highlight some of the questions addressed during the project (called HFRS – the Hackney Family Rights Service), in the hope that these might be of use to other authorities wishing to develop a similar service.

Why is Hackney setting up HFRS?

Five main reasons have been identified:

* The SSD recognises that it holds too much power over families, and it wants to reduce that unequal balance of power. It knows that families do not get enough information about services, are not listened to carefully enough, and are not involved enough in planning meetings and decisions about their children and themselves.
* It recognises that the best decisions are made when families are involved in making plans for their children, and it wants to find ways of involving families more.
* It recognises that services that have been shaped by user views are more likely to be acceptable to users, and it wants to find ways of using families more in the planning and evaluation of services.
* It wants to respond positively to the requirements in the Children Act to consult with children and families about their particular needs.
* It wants to respond to the Act's requirement to consult with the community about services generally.

Who will the service be for?

The project will help children and young people, and adult family members. Family includes the extended family and non-related friends important in the family's life. Individual families will be able to define what family means for them. HFRS will be designed to offer a service to the wide range of ethnic groups in the borough.

Families gaining from the service will include those receiving or wanting services because a child is in need, those involved in child protection procedures, and those with a child looked after by the local authority, either in accommodation or under a court order.

What's going to be on offer?

The project will offer Hackney residents three distinct strands of service:

* independent information, advice and advocacy about their involvement with social services in relation to themselves – if young people – or to their children;
* a place to meet and gain support from others in a similar position to themselves; and
* a way of getting their voice heard in the planning and evaluation of

policies and services provided for children and families. User participation in the design and delivery of policy, procedure and services is wanted to ensure that these are responsive to user needs and promote the best use of resources.

Clarifying some of the essential elements

The work in Hackney and other areas has been guided by the work of FRG and other agencies committed to advocacy work. Part of this work has been to establish some guiding principles about the essential elements of a family advocacy scheme. Current thinking suggests the following:

- Independence – in order to be free of conflicts of interest between service users and providers, the scheme needs to have an independent constitution and management structure from its funders.
- Confidentiality – an understanding that a service user's details will not be passed on to others without that person's permission. An exception would be where a child is clearly at significant risk of harm, but the service user should be given the opportunity to inform social services first.
- Local multi-agency support – which welcomes advocacy as an integral part of quality service provision.
- Advocates to be supported by a paid co-ordinator and administrator. Good advocacy services don't come cheap. They need experienced workers, with a range of languages to meet the needs of service users, sound knowledge of law and practice, and a commitment to enabling users to get their voice heard and their views taken seriously. Advocacy is much more than traditional advice work; the advocate actively promotes somebody's interests and wishes and rights. It is demanding work and requires training, supervision and support. Paid co-ordinators and administrative support should ensure high and continuing standards.
- A commitment to the promotion of equal opportunities and in particular the needs of minority ethnic families, disabled people and lone parents. It is essential that schemes actively promote the interests of all sectors of society, reflected in the constitution of steering groups, the range of advocates recruited, and the style of consultation processes.
- A commitment to the involvement of families from the start. Each scheme needs to be rooted in the perspective of families, not that of professionals. The scheme's starting point must be the difficulties

already experienced by service users, and families' views will be just as valuable as the scheme progresses. They will be best placed to know what works and what doesn't.

COMMENT

Empowerment is about agencies planning services from a user perspective, and then working in partnership with users to meet their defined needs and preferred solutions. For local authorities, the central challenge of the Children Act 1989 was to work out ways of bolstering a family's own efforts to provide well for their children, and to replace punitive notions of rescuing children from unsuitable homes with the more positive practice of supporting parents through periods of crisis.

The required shift in emphasis, from targeted services for children at risk of abuse, towards universal provision of family support services intended to reduce stress and state intervention, has been uncomfortable and slow for most local authorities. But where the problems have been acknowledged, small gains are being made. Hard-pressed but committed authorities are finding ways to increase their budget for family support work, to appoint dedicated family support managers, to consult with users, and to encourage the development of schemes that give a voice to children and families who have traditionally had little help in getting themselves heard and taken seriously.

Family group conferences and family advocacy schemes provide two modest, but important, ways of adjusting the balance of power between agencies and service users.

REFERENCES

Berridge, D. and Cleaver, H. (1987) *Foster Home Breakdown*, Oxford: Blackwell.
Department of Social Welfare (1989) *Practice Paper – Family Decision Making*, Staff Briefing Paper, Cm 34, Wellington, New Zealand: Department of Social Welfare.
FRG (Family Rights Group) (1990) *Getting Going . . . Tips for Starting a Local Support Group*, London: Family Rights Group.
—— (1991) *The Work of Self-Help Groups for Families With Children in Care*, London: Family Rights Group.
—— (1995) *Family Advocacy News* (quarterly bulletins).
Fisher, M., Marsh, P., Phillips, D. and Sainsbury, E. (1986) *In and Out of Care*, London: Batsford.
Fruin, D. and Vernon, J. (1986) *In Care – A Study of Social Work Decision Making*, London: National Children's Bureau.
Hassall, I. and Maxwell, G. (1991) 'The Family Group Conference', in Hassall,

I. (ed.), *An Appraisal of the First Year of the Children, Young Persons and their Families Act 1989*, Wellington, New Zealand: Office of the Commissioner for Children.

Holman, R. (1991) 'Friday, sent the girl to borrow two slices of bread . . .', *Guardian Society*, 12 June.

Hosie, K. (1985) *A proposal for setting up a support group for parents of children in care*, Totnes: Dartington Social Research Unit.

McGowan, B. (1977) 'Case advocacy – a study of the intervention process in case advocacy', in C. Grosser, (ed.), *New Directions in Community Organising*, New York: Praeger Publishers.

Millham, S., Bullock, R., Hosie, K. and Haak, M. (1986) *Lost in Care: The Problems of Maintaining Links Between Children in Care and their Families*, Aldershot: Gower.

Millham, S., Bullock, R., Hosie, K. and Little, M. (1989) *Access Disputes in Child Care*, Aldershot: Gower.

Monaco, M. and Thoburn, J. (1987) *Self-help for Parents With Children in Care*, Department of Social Work Monograph, University of East Anglia.

Parents' Aid (1991) *A Guide for Families – Your Child and Social Services*, Harlow: Parents Aid.

Plant, R. (1970) *Social and Moral Theory in Casework*, London: Routledge and Kegan Paul.

Wolfensberger, W. (1977) *A Global Multi-Component Advocacy Protection Scheme*, Monograph, Canadian Association for the Mentally Retarded, 4700 Keele Street, Downsview, Toronto, Ontario, Canada.

Chapter 9

Long-term development

Neighbourhood community development work on estates

Barry Hulyer

This chapter describes the work of a community development project working on two south-coast outlying estates since 1983. The project is, as described by David Thomas (1983), a 'neighbourhood project' working to a community development model. Thomas argued for developing teams of community workers, based in neighbourhoods, as the way forward.

I came to the project because I wanted to work in a neighbourhood. I wanted to put what I saw as the important theories of community development to the test, and I wanted to do it on an estate. Either I wanted this because I enjoyed most these fieldwork placements on my community work course, or because of experience of the imperfections when I worked for a centrally-based community resource centre or because I grew up on a council estate myself. I mention this because I believe that, just as community members need to be motivated to get involved and the worker needs a good idea of what those are, the worker needs also to understand their own motivations.

I believe that this motivation needs to be accompanied by a strong belief system, not only to succeed as a neighbourhood community development worker, but to survive. I hope that this account will show why.

THE BEGINNING – EXISTING ON A SHOE-STRING

I came to the project in 1984 to take up a single worker post. The project is an independent voluntary organisation and only had enough money for six months into the future. There was no team of workers, as in Thomas's model, although today we have nine staff (six full-time equivalents). The effects of being a single worker seeking to respond to various expressed needs should not be underestimated. I have seen many workers try to survive in similar situations and I can honestly say that the ones who have, did what I managed to do – draw in other people so you're not on your own. There's always someone; a social worker with a few hours (rare these days I admit), job-creation trainees, students on placement, local community volunteers – they can all perform useful functions. I even collared my personal friends – 'I'll buy you a few pints if you'll help me deliver some leaflets beforehand!' I also found it invaluable to draw in support; professional, experienced advice, encouragement and help, from people I will always be indebted to.

All this support was necessary, not only because of the demanding nature of community work and helping me to link theory with my practice, but mainly because the project was broke! We always existed on a shoe-string and often were not able to afford that! In the early days we started a financial year with under 50 per cent of the year's budget. Twice, only loans from wealthy contacts, made through the supporters mentioned earlier, kept us going till the next grant.

There were benefits which arose from our continual financial un-certainty – it ensured that, however we could manage it, groups we set up had the capacity to survive on their own, because they were going to have to any minute. Our impoverishment forced us into good practice. Good practice is, in community development work, essential to achieving good outcomes. Good practice is, I believe, recognised and developed through our values and beliefs.

VALUES AND BELIEFS

The values and beliefs which should underpin community development practice are described in many books (Thomas 1983; Twelvetrees 1982) and more coherently than I could manage. I would like to emphasise that for me, the concepts of 'working from the bottom up' ('bubble up' rather than 'trickle down') and 'starting from where people are at' need to be far more than just words for the effective community development worker. We have to really believe in them and show it through our practice, then the people whom we work with will believe in us. We need to show that we respect the people we work with and we believe in their capacities (and if we don't, we can't show it).

We need to internalise the concepts so that we start with ourselves. We need to start from where we are at and take fully on board the feminist concept that 'the personal is political'.

In line with another of my 'little rules' that says we should not expect community members to do what we ourselves wouldn't (and show it by our actions), if we are expecting people to change and grow, we have to accept that we must also.

One of the better places to start is with language and communication. We need to be clear. We need to speak simply. We need to avoid the use of jargon and other forms of speech that exclude. As Twelvetrees says, 'We can train ourselves to become aware of the words we use.'

COMMUNITY DEVELOPMENT IN PRACTICE – INTANGIBLE GAINS

Let's look at what the project has achieved over the last twelve years, starting with the intangibles, the way community development can affect the participants. Twelvetrees describes it as follows:

Community Development encourages people to take positive action and to believe that they can act, that they can cause change, which can sometimes help to give their lives greater meaning. Of the lessons learned by the participants in community action perhaps the most important are new attitudes, new political perspectives and a broader understanding of how the world works.

(Twelvetrees 1982: 44)

and for Thomas,

Task and process are locked in a virtuous circle: when people are effective in community action they acquire a sense of their own ability and power, and enhance their understanding and competence. This helps to make them feel more confident, more positive about themselves, more capable. This in turn makes it more likely that they will engage in further community activity and thus improve their lot, and that of others.

(Thomas 1983: 129)

I can honestly say that I have seen the effects described above in our communities. Some active participants have changed radically, both within themselves and in their material situations. Jenny was a housewife with four children and a working husband (in a low-income job), they were struggling, but getting by. Now Jenny has paid work herself in another community on a children's project. She learned a great deal of her skills from her voluntary involvement in her own community, starting on a summer playscheme, through a festival group, on through the project's management committee, etc. There are many other examples.

I have also seen the process of community organisation change the way people feel about themselves and where they live. When I started with the project I spent a great deal of time listening to people talk about their community and asking how they felt about it. Typical responses were:

'They should knock down all these houses and start again.'
'Everybody here is so apathetic.'
'I just wanna move, I'm on the transfer list.'
'You'll never get anybody here to do anything to help themselves or anybody else, mate.'

and my favourite, when I asked what should be done with the old building in the park, 'Bomb it!'

Now that old building is covered by a beautiful mural, painted, a wall each by: young children, older children, young people and the adults from the flats round the park. Also, following a 'Plan for the Park', created by local people, the building will be redeveloped into a café and play-base for children.

I rarely hear such talk of desperation to leave now, although I am sure it still exists. One young mother, new to the area, told me recently when I asked the old favourite about what she thought of the estate, 'Yeah, it's good, I asked to be moved here.' I nearly fell off my chair and just restrained myself from shouting 'you did what!!' I have to be honest and say that we (the community and the project), may have achieved improvements but there can't be many people that would say that (although one has to consider that the extent of her choice was between one housing estate or another). However, a number of community members tell me that they are now proud to live here.

I don't believe this sort of change can be achieved only through tangible improvements, or even the intangibles. I have learned that we have to use the media, and other external organisations, to promote the good things about the area, sometimes in quite indirect ways. An example is the community festival. When I started working with this group I cannot say that I foresaw what an impact they would have. Through large-scale spectacular shows the festival appeared on the front pages of all the local newspapers and on TV news. I remember one letter to the local paper (written by a councillor) wholeheartedly praising the event, which finished with 'they have dragged this town into the 20th Century'. I admit I felt good reading that – imagine what the local community members felt, not only those 150 involved in organising the event, but everyone else too.

This is giving the area a more positive image. I am frequently contacted by the media in their quest for stories and often I help them and together we promote positive events, but just as often they will ask things like 'what's the drug problem like in the area?' I reply 'oh, average, about the same as anywhere else!' Not many headlines in that reply, so no story appears. In fact, some major funds are realised for prevention work and we get these because of the statistics on drug use in the area we can present. I can imagine people reading this and thinking that I'm manipulating the press and consequently the local community. I will answer that charge. Going back to the importance of positive image, and how community members now view the area, relating it to Thomas's statement about people feeling 'more confident, more positive about themselves, more capable', surely the media 'feeding them' this image is good. There is surely no virtue in people feeling miserable. If the alternative is the media creating negative images of the community and its members (which I could collude with) then it is likely that people will feel miserable. I think the women's movement has already taught us about how the media has this effect – for 'women's body image' read 'people's community image'. I feel that as community workers we can often make grave mistakes in this area. We need to recognise the difference between the 'poverty and problems' which need to be emphasised to funders and the positive images which recognise local people's achievements.

We have all seen articles in community newspapers saying 'where are you, there are thousands receive this paper and if you don't turn up to this or that we're going to shut that or this down!' It never makes me feel very inspired. It certainly doesn't make me think 'I'll mosey on down there, they sound like a fun bunch!' I realise that the people who write like this feel demoralised but is it likely to encourage others to respond? Obviously, I've learnt something from the 1980s – image; it's crucial and we've got to create it before someone creates it for us!

TANGIBLE AND CONCRETE IMPROVEMENTS

If we look at tangibles, what has the community created with a bit of help from the project? What can twelve years of sustained, unreconstructed community development actually achieve in a neighbourhood?

In the case of this project it has achieved the creation of over ninety different community groups. Not all still exist; some died through lack of funding, some disbanded having achieved their aims, some turned into something else and some of them just plain failed. A good deal do still exist, and some of them are as old as the project. When groups are that old its likely that perhaps none, or only a few, of the original members are still involved. One of the benefits of long-term neighbourhood community development work is that there is still an organisation for them to ask for assistance when things go wrong. I've worked with groups who have been totally independent for years and I've not even been to a meeting for three or four years and suddenly they come to me because they've got dangerously low on numbers, or whatever. Sometimes they will tell me how they feel, I'll listen, tell them I think their plans to rectify the situation are excellent and they then solve their own problems. Other times it leads to the project working intensively with them for another six months or so. Even in the former case it is possible that they may not have had just enough confidence to carry on if the project wasn't here – just to give a bit of encouragement.

These ninety different groups may sound impressive but the vast majority of them are not particularly innovative or different. They are the community's ideas. They include playgroups, playschemes, after-school clubs, community newspapers, youth clubs, tenants'/residents' associations, community associations, elderly persons' lunch clubs, community festival, advice groups, children's circus, drama groups, social clubs, mural projects, youth adventure group, youth newspaper.

Our work has led to the creation of thirteen full-time jobs and around sixty-one part-time jobs, but I do not believe this is a useful or helpful basis for evaluation of the work, or worth adopting as an aim. I can also calculate investment into the estates of over £3,000,000 resulting from the project's existence, but again, that is 'small beer' when considered against one health service or local authority building costing a similar sum.

Included in that sum of money, and often identified as the most tangible and concrete improvements that have been achieved, are two community buildings. We have helped community members, through the organisation of two community associations for the estates, to design, fund and build a community centre for each.

The first was purpose built, and entirely funded by the borough council (but not until quite a fight/campaign had been waged), and the second took three years to raise the £350,000 that it needed. This is again a point where one has to recognise that our 1970s style unreconstructed community development work was tinted by the mores of the 1980s. The project fundraised the £350,000 having agreed a contract with the community association for a 7.5 per cent fundraising fee. Not an arrangement that I would have contemplated in the 1970s but with a touch of the Saul Alinsky's about it (see Alinsky 1972). Alinsky was the

American activist behind the Industrial Areas Foundation who required communities to pay him and his 'activists' to go into an area, thus guaranteeing 'commitment', he believed.

The situation then in 1989 was that an association of local community members were needing £350,000. The project had fundraising experience, but was still desperately insolvent itself and needed to find a new source of money. Without the project what would happen to the community's plans (worked on with a sympathetic architect) for a central resource and focal point for their community? The project raised the money, kept itself solvent for four years on its fee, and the building was opened in 1993.

I would not advise workers and organisations to enter into these arrangements with community groups unless there is a very good relationship between the parties already existing. There needs to be complete trust and belief in each other, going beyond a simple written contract. There is a good deal of scope for misunderstandings, mistrust and disagreement which, between a neighbourhood development organisation and the major representative community organisation in that neighbourhood, would be so serious as to make continued work in the area probably impossible. However, if the relationship is good and secure then there are obvious advantages for both parties which can strengthen future relationships, as our experience has shown.

WORK WITH YOUNG PEOPLE IN THE COMMUNITY

One development of the project's is, perhaps, innovative. It's certainly difficult to find examples of similar practice elsewhere in the UK to learn from. I refer to the blending of our basic community development practice with detached youth work. This is a style of youth work, so called because it is not based in a building. The youth workers spend a part of their time seeking out young people where they congregate; on the streets, in parks, outside shopping parades, in cafés and pubs, etc. Where we differ from more purist detached youth work is that the youth workers also work to the basic aims and objectives of the project, set in 1984 and unchanged. They are:

1 Assist and support existing community groups and work with local residents to initiate new groups capable of responding to identified needs.
2 Liaise between statutory agencies and voluntary groups to promote

community resources for the area and work together on common priorities.
3 Promote the development of community buildings, managed by the community, providing facilities for all residents.
4 Encourage participation in all forms of voluntary activity and offer support, encouragement and training to those volunteers.

A purist detached youth work point of view is that whilst it is possible that the need for new youth groups and activities may arise from detached or 'streetwork', it should not be the same workers that seek to meet these needs. Indeed, in that model, the young people may not even be involved in meeting the need at all – another agency may do it. The rationale behind this is that it will draw the detached youth workers away from 'streetwork' into project work and it is this counselling and advocacy that is the main aim of the work. Whilst our youth workers are involved in helping young people on an individual basis with various problems they encounter – drugs, family break-up, unemployment, homelessness, etc. – it is our main (community development) aim to encourage them to respond to their situation collectively. We believe that they too can benefit from the intangibles mentioned earlier.

I have to say that whilst community development theory is simple and easy to understand as a concept, it is not at all easy to practise (many widely differing skills are required) and to do it with young people is even more difficult and time consuming. I believe the key is in matching the strategies employed to the developmental stages of the young people themselves and I will explore this in more depth later on.

Our youth work, over four and a half years, has resulted in the development of many new groups and activities, controlled largely or wholly by young people themselves. These are again not radical. Groups include: young people's newspaper, young mums' group, adventure group, sports groups, youth coffee bar, music group, motorbike group, sexual health information group, fantasy games group, etc.

This style of work is difficult not only because of the age of the participants but also because of the way those participants are sometimes viewed by the wider (adult) community. It is difficult for them to gain access to meeting space because of fears that they will 'smash the place up'. Though why a group of young people should go to all the trouble of forming a constituted community group just to smash somewhere up, beats me! They could just break in to do that.

Difficulties between young people and adults on estates is not, of course, unusual. We have, however, had some hopeful signs that our neighbourhood-based team, which now includes both youth workers and community workers, can have positive effects upon these fractious relationships. I will recount two recent experiences, not radical or particularly innovative, but they are starting to show interesting results. The results may be because of the length of time we have worked in the area and the new 'culture and belief' – what Thomas (1983) terms 'community coherence'.

The first example arose when I answered the phone to a somewhat distraught woman resident who said:

> Look I don't know if you can help, I've tried everyone else I could think of, we're going mad here, the police are useless, social services suggested I ring you. I know you work with community groups so you probably can't help!

She went on to describe how she lived next to a small green where 'teenagers' congregated at night and made her and her neighbours' lives 'a complete misery'. The young people apparently took drugs, drank strong alcohol and threw the cans and bottles in the road and their front yards, lit fires, had 'full sex between the parked cars', were making 'molotov' cocktails to throw at them because they complained and even poisoned her neighbour's goldfish! She, and her neighbours, were obviously frightened for their young children and themselves and gave the impression of living in a sort of 'curfew' situation. As I talked to her it became clear that she and her neighbours were in constant communication and even had a small meeting to discuss the situation in one of their houses. Interesting then, I thought, that she perceived the project as working with 'groups' and didn't see herself as already involved in any sort of collective action!

I tentatively suggested that if they wanted to hold another meeting one of our community workers could attend and find out more about the situation. She was overjoyed, but I had to 'back-peddle' and stress that we could not promise to do anything that would improve the situation.

The community development worker who was responsible for that area within our team was fairly inexperienced, only having been with us for two months. She was apprehensive about 'walking into the lion's den' and I couldn't say that I blamed her. I restrained myself from going to support her. I felt the residents would probably have automatically responded to me as the person with the answers (and a man!) and that would restrict her capacity to build a relationship with them. I think I was right! When we discussed this first meeting I advised her to take it very slowly, just to listen and to recognise that the residents were going to need time to 'get it off their chests' and to feel that someone was taking their concern seriously. The worker met with the group (of about twelve residents) weekly after that and the 'getting it off their chests' stage took about eight weeks. The worker got a policeman to come and listen to their grievances, although they still don't feel the police actually did anything.

Meanwhile, starting the day after the phone call, two of our detached youth workers started to visit 'the green' on their streetwork sessions. They soon made contact with the group of 'teenagers' who turned out to be a mixed-gender group of about twelve, aged from 13 years to 18 years, all hanging out together. This was quite unusual in itself. They felt the adults persecuted them and that they only responded aggressively because they wouldn't leave them alone. They were all hanging around the green because the older ones were afraid to leave the immediate area because they were being seriously bullied by other kids on the estate (there was an incident with an iron bar). The youth workers discovered they would be happy to meet somewhere else occasionally if they had somewhere 'safe' to go. The workers talked to the vicar of a church hall who agreed they could meet there weekly, on a temporary basis, for free. The workers met with the group for about six or seven weeks. They helped them to start organising trips away from the area for themselves; ten-pin bowling, ice-skating, etc. The workers also encouraged them to think about how the residents experienced their behaviour.

Meanwhile, the adults, with the community development worker's help, had decided to start a residents' association and, separately, a neighbourhood watch scheme – they had earlier been thinking more along the lines of a vigilante group! The worker was able, after they'd collectively calmed down a bit, to help them discuss what life was like for teenagers these days; they had assumed it was the same as when they were growing up. They had not come to terms with the 'no jobs/no home/no future' generation. After a while one of the residents, who has a large shed/cabin thing in their garden, let the kids use it when it was raining. I met with the group once, when they wanted some advice about their inaugural public meeting, and they were a very amiable, positive group by then. What an excellent job both the community development worker and the detached youth workers did. To do this, though, requires an enormous amount of communication and sharing of information, quite difficult for the workers.

In May 1995, on VE Day, the residents' association held a street party on 'the green'. The young people organised several stalls and decorated the green for the event. The young people earned money from stalls which they use to finance their 'trips'. Leading up to the event the two groups held several joint planning meetings – they all sat down together in the same room! So, although this was quite a basic piece of work, I think the adults and the young people have experienced it as a major change in their lives.

The other piece of work, which developed along similar lines, arose out of young people's use of motorbikes in the area. The estates are on the furthest edge of the conurbation and lie alongside the South Downs. A lot of the young people own cheap, badly maintained, usually illegal, off-road motorbikes. Residents were getting very upset about the young people 'racing' them up and down the only straight road on the estate and they were constantly in trouble with the police for riding them on farmland and nature reserves on the Downs. Things were definitely 'coming to a head' and so the youth workers held meetings to ascertain the young people's views on the situation. The meetings were attended by thirty-five young people, aged 14 to 18 years. Do young people happily attend 'boring meetings' because of the 'community coherence' that has been built up I wonder, or does it happen like this everywhere?

This work progressed much like the earlier example, except in this case the youth workers asked the young people if they could find adults who would support them in working towards a more positive situation. Six months later the Kickstart Motorbike Group was formed, with a committee of twelve adults, and forty junior members. The group is seeking to develop an off-road motorbike track. A youth worker and a community development worker work closely with the group but so far we have been unable to find a suitable site. Meanwhile the group organises regular trips away from the area for biking and also maintenance workshops for young people and is building a good reputation for itself.

These developments do not function without problems between the young people and the adults but they do show improvement. I would not have felt confident about our capacity to achieve these results in the early days of the project and feel they have in some sense been made possible by the more 'coherent community', and in part because of the community's growing trust and faith in the project itself.

CHILDREN AND FAMILIES

Children and families are the theme of this book and so now I will concentrate on what long-term community development work has, and can, do for them. I will concentrate on children (and young people).

Obviously, the development of after-school clubs, summer playschemes, new playgroups, etc., which we have been involved in have benefited children (as well as their parents). Equally it can be seen that community associations, residents' associations and a community festival can benefit children and families through improving the area generally, or the housing.

These are the tangible benefits but how do children benefit from the intangible? The area, historically, has a high incidence of children on the 'at risk' register or in care; whilst numbers are still fairly high they have steadily been going down. I must point out that during the last ten years social services have changed the way they administer these cases and that may account for some of the decrease but I believe that the project's work also accounts for it and so do social services managers. If community members are being empowered in the ways described by Thomas (1983) and Twelvetrees (1982) and some of them are social services clients, then it seems reasonable to assume that their new-found confidence and self-belief will help them avoid the stressful situations that lead to, for example, physical abuse of their children. Whilst true for individuals I believe it is true also for the community collectively. If collectively the community has a more positive image of itself this should affect their culture, expectations and beliefs. With regard to the position of, and treatment of children within the community, I certainly see fewer naked 4-year-olds wandering the streets at 10.00pm.

By working in the area for twelve years I have seen the effects upon children of parents involving themselves in community organising. Just like it often seems that children of councillors often become councillors, then children who have grown up experiencing their parents involved in collective action seem to view it as a more 'natural' activity themselves as they grow up – perhaps this is what we experience in our work with young people.

One criticism that is levelled at community development work, however, is that of 'the danger of community workers using children as a means of getting at the adults rather than as people in their own right' (Hasler, 1995: 180).

I think the project is not immune to this criticism and have been considering it seriously recently. I have come to the conclusion that in our situation, as a generalist community development organisation that does not concentrate on specialist, intensive work with children, we can consider the developmental stage of the child or young person and offer a greater level of involvement, participation and decision making to the child as it gets older. It sounds simple, but it requires skill in recognising the child's stage in development. This is easier if you've known the child for a while and watched them grow up – another benefit of long-term work.

In practice this means simply ensuring that a young child, or group of children is actually asked about what they want out of a particular development – they are consulted just as an adult should be. I recall suggesting to the project management committee that if we were to accept the role of fundraiser for an infant school interested in re-developing its grounds, we should insist that we undertake a community consultation into the plans drawn up by an architect and the school governors. I was asked who we would consult and replied 'the parents, the teachers, the local community and the children who will use the grounds'. A councillor present was appalled, 'the children! They are only 5 years old for goodness sake!' I think a younger, more inexperienced me wouldn't have suggested it either, but through years of thinking always of participation, involvement and empowerment it has at last started to permeate all areas of my thoughts and practice. Of course, the children have the capacity to decide what they like and dislike in their playground, their environment and their life.

When, in 1990, we undertook a consultation about what the community wanted from their local park, we asked children of all ages, young people and adults. The 5 to 7 year-olds came up with almost exactly the same answers as the 8 to 12 year-olds, the 13 to 20 year-olds and most of the adults – a levelled area for playing football, reducing dogs' mess, somewhere to buy ice creams, etc. When children are a bit older (say after-school club age) they can happily devise most of a programme of events understanding financial restraints.

But when are young people old enough to take control of their own activities entirely? Of course there isn't a set age when anyone is ready for responsibility and power, it differs with different young people and the skill lies in identifying it. Generally, though, I would argue that it is earlier than most of our society thinks. We have made mistakes in this area and are still learning.

We recently agreed to undertake a joint initiative with another agency involving a group of young people who wanted to set up an unspecified activity. One of the difficulties with this interagency working is that practising community development work must involve constant evaluation as the process develops. The plan must change as the situation changes and the participants more clearly identify their needs and desires. This is more difficult and cumbersome when it needs constant inter-agency meetings to agree changes. We didn't communicate enough and although both parties agreed with the young people that we would help them set up their own coffee bar, it didn't happen.

When our two agencies met to discuss the deadlock and consider a different approach, I soon realised that there was a mismatch with the young people's development stage; they couldn't actually run it themselves. It would appear that at the first meeting the young people identified the need and pledged themselves to learning to run the coffee bar. The group included older, more capable young people who didn't attend subsequent meetings. Both the project and the other agency carried on regardless with the original plan. Clearly there was a failure to consider the developmental capacity of the young people. It became inevitable that the idea should be abandoned or someone should offer to run it for the young people. This was not our 'brief' and the other agency didn't have the capacity. So a group of young people were left feeling let down. I think it should be a major rule of neighbourhood development work that we shouldn't let people down – it doesn't lead to confident, optimistic communities. It's not the end of the world though, as long as we learn from it and groups are, in general, enjoying success and achievement in their neighbourhood.

Our other work with 16 to 25 year-olds does show that a community development model can work and young people can empower themselves, if they are given the opportunity.

We could obviously improve our practice with children and young people and I have seriously reconsidered my practice since reading Peter Newell (1995). I would urge others to read it!

WHAT COMMUNITY DEVELOPMENT CANNOT ACHIEVE

There are many other issues I do not believe a community development organisation like ours can address, with both adults and children.

When it comes to children, there are some whose needs we have singularly failed to meet, the group I refer to is 'the little terrors', for want of a better title. In one estate there is a group of no more than five or six children whose behaviour causes considerable pain and anguish to most of the rest of the community. I'm sure you can imagine them already! I first noticed they were going to be a serious problem when they were 6 or 7 years old (they're 11 or 12 now). They vandalise things (quite seriously), they steal, they bully the other kids, they disrupt the community's attempt to provide activities for the other children and they appear to react to any adult who talks to them, however nicely and sympathetically (even me!) with a stream of vitriolic abuse. When a child of around 8 years reacts to a very liberal, kindly lady of 70 years who says 'Please don't throw stones through my window, I just can't afford to mend it again, feel free to play here though and I'll get you some lemonade if you'd like', with 'I'm gonna take those big tits of yours and squeeze them till they spurt milk into the air and then make you drink it', then I think we need to be concerned about what is happening to that child.

The agencies that seem to have some responsibility, social services, schools, the police, etc., don't seem to be worried enough to do anything to help them (despite my attempts to suggest they might). We all know these 'terrors' exist, the Home Secretary knows (he wants to lock them all up) and the schools certainly know – they are sooner or later almost permanently excluded from education. It makes me feel very sad and angry. No one needs education and support more than these kids.

The present situation costs us very dearly as a community, and as a society. I have watched two or three 'waves' of these children grow up and it seems inevitable that their behaviour grows ever more unacceptable to the rest of us until we, and they, pay the highest price, that of detention in Her Majesty's prisons.

I would propose a simple, relatively cheap and seemingly obvious solution. At the youngest age when it becomes clear they are going beyond the boundaries adhered to by the other children – hopefully 6 or 7 years old – they receive some undivided attention. I would like to see a small team of professionals, including a social worker, a child therapist and perhaps a children's community worker, offer them whatever it takes to make them join a small group just for them. Not labelling them 'clients' would help gain their parents' acceptance. This team would just go and hang out where the kids are and show some real interest in them. I believe the children would respond.

The reason I believe this would bring results is that occasionally we have achieved a level of involvement with one of these 'little terrors' that has led to a complete change in their behaviour. I want to emphasise that I am not talking about the quite large numbers of children whose life is enhanced by, and behaviour changed by community involvement in after-school clubs, etc. I'm talking about the kids who are barred from everything very quickly because no one can handle them – certainly not volunteers or playworkers paid £3.75 an hour!

If they were worked with intensively, and in an unstigmatised way, given support while they were still so young it would surely have a similar effect to the example I can remember of a 15 year old. He wasn't one of the worst but by his own recent admission he was heading for 'trouble' and wasn't expecting much future. It was a fluke he became interested in a video project I was involved with and it was an even bigger fluke that the first time he seriously overstepped the boundaries of the group I said the right thing to keep him involved whilst maintaining the boundaries. He's 22 years old now; an artist and a journalist. He lives out of the area but comes back to help the summer festival every year.

I would hope that as social services starts to move away from its over-concentration on child protection, as it now appears to be doing, it would consider itself a mover in such developments. If social services wish to listen to the voices of users (even those who are not yet users) surely no one can be speaking more plainly and, yes, loudly, than these children, through their actions.

In passing I would like to touch on a need we have been aware of for years but unable to meet. Namely a fund to pay for parents' child care, mainly women, who are unable to engage themselves fully in their community due to child care responsibilities. We work in an area with high numbers of single parents and many of these are clearly unable, for example, to attend an evening meeting – a few pounds would pay for a babysitter and enable them to experience the empowering nature of collective action. Alas, no funder we have found has so far been willing to finance such a scheme.

CONCLUSION

Community development is a long-term process. In general it takes longer to teach someone else to do something than it does to do it yourself. It's a long process because each group that a community development worker works with takes a long time to develop autonomy, if it's done properly. Each group needs clear aims, as many people as possible involved, an efficient structure, a few early successes, etc., if it is to survive and prosper. Most importantly, though, all the participants must be fully aware that it is their group and they are going to run it. I believe a worker should never start or run a group/activity themselves hoping that the community will take it over later. This is without doubt the biggest mistake that I have witnessed workers, including myself, make.

I have learnt that in neighbourhood work it is best to start small – to help people with small, achievable things that will succeed. Success breeds success – and creates optimism. Success and optimism are vital to build the confidence which we call empowerment. We cannot empower other people, they must empower themselves. This is best described in an old joke:

'*How many psychiatrists does it take to change a light-bulb?*'
'Only one, but the light-bulb has to want to change!'

If the project has been successful it's only because the community has. All those individuals who have done the really hard work have empowered themselves, we are just here to support them.

I believe that if we are to create Thomas's 'coherent communities' (1983) we must concentrate on the small things and do them well. The whole picture will take care of itself if all the small parts are compatible to the whole. For community development work this is where the beliefs, the value system and the theory become important. This should underpin all our work. If we are really true to the values then there is a very good chance that the optimistic, confident, positive community will emerge. I would liken it to the development of a photograph. If we concentrate on all the small mechanics of the process, ensuring it is in focus, etc., then a photograph of perfect clarity will emerge from the developing tray.

So after twelve years I feel that the project, working in partnership with the community, has helped to achieve this desired 'coherent community' to a certain extent. I feel there is still a way to go and more to be achieved before these estates could be described as a good place to live.

If the project were not here tomorrow I believe that the longer term, more ambitious ideas the community has identified would probably not come to fruition without professional support. Whilst I am sure that some professional support would be available, it would be either from a generalist support agency which covers a much wider area or from a specialist worker only mandated to support certain initiatives (play, under-5's, etc.). I do not believe that either, or both, of these interventions, however valuable, would provide the in-depth sort of support that a wide range of small grassroots community organisations needs. I think that the culture of confidence and belief would suffer.

I believe that Thomas's 'neighbourhood community development teams', operating in small, deprived, geographical areas, practising unreconstructed community development work (but adapted to the 1990s), are as necessary now as when he wrote about them thirteen years ago. For this to happen we principally need two things. The first is, of course, proper long-term funding for community development work. That means funding which recognises that communities should decide for themselves what will best regenerate their areas, instead of the ridiculous overemphasis on exact targets (how many people? etc.) that prevails presently. The second is more community development work training. There are too few community work courses and there needs to be post-qualifying training for social workers and other professionals in development work, as it seems obvious that the implementation of the Community Care Act and the Children Act requires them.

REFERENCES

Alinsky, S. 1969. *'Reveille for Radicals'*, New York: Vintage Books.
Alinsky, S. 1972. *'Rules for Radicals'*, New York: Vintage Books.
Hasler, J. 1995. 'Belonging and Becoming: The Child Growing up in the Community', in P. Henderson (ed.), *'Children and Communities'*, London: Pluto Press.
Newell, P. 1995. 'Rights, Participation and Neighbourhoods', in P. Henderson (ed.), *'Children and Communities'*, London: Pluto Press.
Thomas, D. 1983. *'The Making of Community Work'*, London: George Allen & Unwin.
Twelvetrees, A. 1982. *'Community Work'*, Basingstoke: Macmillan Education.

Chapter 10

Think global, act local

Towards residents' control of their life, health and environment – tools and skills in social development in France

Marie-Renée Bourget-Daitch and Chris Warren

This is an account of interventions by a social development team, a local training and development initiative assembled by MDSL-Formation (MDSL 1995), a French national community development agency. MDSL works alongside local people to establish development projects born out of the needs of local people and within a framework of partnership, based on the theme of 'Adults and parents and their neighbourhoods'.

MDSL-Formation comprises fieldworkers, academics and trainers who have worked in the field of social work, public health or in local development for several years (development workers, social workers, doctors in public and community health, architects, educationalists, sociologists, anthropologists and psychologists).

In this chapter four tools of development are discussed using local project examples, in which we discover an encouraging solidarity in theory and practice intervention which matches with other chapters in this book. We underline the model of the development-training team, carefully establishing its local mandate, recruiting a variety of team members with relevant technical skills, and holding firmly to the principle of 'act local, think global'.

NETWORK DEVELOPMENT

The idea of network development grew in France around 1980–81. In the domain of social and community work, the concept drew partly on American practices and theories of network family therapy (Speck and Attneave 1973) and partly on the experience of Quebecois researchers and social workers as part of community development. Networkers are also inspired by the practices of the Brazilian Paulo Freire (1972). They seek to rebuild social links, enable the definition of needs at local level to contribute to an appropriate service response, and allow a better collective awareness of the economic, cultural and social contradictions in which individuals and communities are involved.

Since 1985 the network concept has been widely used in many different contexts. Joel de Rosnay explains how, in a world where communications have become so intensified and often entangled, there is a place for the creation of networks to

> ensure a continuity between the micro and the macro. This 'capillarisation' of networks allows everyone to be in contact with other networks. We want to send out information to take part more directly in the running of those large systems in which we are elements and which currently leads us towards the development of horizontal links.
>
> (Rosnay 1984)

Networking is not a technique that is learnt; it is an art of living. In the face of the complexity of the system, networking provides a means of bringing projects to fruition, of feeling tied to and part of a set of values and interests on many different levels. It means that anonymity, isolation and depression may be avoided. This type of open network

> is made outside established institutions, where people organise themselves in order to change something together in a non-bureaucratic manner. Its strength comes from widespread acceptance by its constituent elements of mutual reward systems, and of solidarity which reinforces its coherence.
>
> (Rosnay 1984)

However, the use of the network as a tool of social development in a community must entail a certain number of ethical rules without which it can be a tool of powerful manipulation. You can provoke, induce, create a network from the inside, never from the outside as an expert. Knowledge about a population must never mean its manipulation so that a need is created for a network . That is why in the early stages of the exercise, the expression 'network practice' only makes sense when used about endogenous practices in a stable population where there are existing networks and where networks need to be developed. It means working alongside people so that they can find their own solutions to problems, to help them to 'rediscover knowledge', even those who do not believe they have any. This requires a range of skills which cannot be acquired except in a permanent exchange of 'know-how'.

If we are to escape from the idea of a hierarchical organisation where the few decide what is best for the whole structure – or the charisma of some becomes a point of reference for the rest, or again the responsibility of one or some prevents the others from taking full part in the construction of a coherent whole – it is essential to put in place a flexible structure, which should be as far as possible horizontal, where each person shares her thoughts, questions, knowledge gained, experiences, without fear of being judged but with the obligation of holding herself responsible.

It is for this reason that MDSL-Formation is trying to put into place a structure based on the network model, where each is responsible for her work and her workshops, but at the same time, each person is connected to all the others, to exchange, share, ask for help and offer it. Around each workshop there is a network, informal at first becoming formal later, made up of skills, commonalities and opportunities. No one should work alone. Once or twice a year, development training is offered to all the workers so that little by little a common spirit is created around the ethic of intervention.

Each of the development projects activated by MDSL-Formation relies on a network of professionals and/or local inhabitants who live or work on the project's territory. The aim is that the search for a solution to the problems identified and the construction of the projects themselves will be supported at the core by a group of people who have a commonality of interests. The work of the network spreads and takes on many different forms. Around MDSL-Formation, a network of medical/ social professionals meets and exchanges practical skills between French *départements* and between countries such as Switzerland, Canada and Brazil.

Case study 1 – Pause Bien Être (Rouen)

Community Networking – a tool in social development

A women's group emerged from a long-term initiative called 'Insertion, Development' (district of Rouen) which involved residents who were either on *RMI*-benefit linked to re-entry into work – or who were unemployed on a long-term basis in Rouen. The group was organised in the district through the work conducted by the local nursery teacher and some of the women. MDSL-Formation was thereafter made known to the group who gave themselves the name of *Pause Bien Être*. It was then able to be enrolled in a programme called 'Réseau InterSite Santé'

(RISS – inter-project health network) which MDSL-Formation pilots in association with others.

At first, six women, all mothers between 22 and 42 years old, some of whom were already known to the PMI (Protection Maternelle et Infantile) through the nursery teacher, met on a weekly basis, emerging from their isolation, finding a place, a space to talk, relax and share their main concerns. (For example, two of them have children with severe disabilities and find it difficult to be recognised not only as valid negotiators but also as mothers with skills.)

An MDSL-Formation development worker agreed to track the group and its progress, helping it in its early stages in order to establish recognition. At the same time people and resources are brought together and, with the group's agreement, they are made available to bring in the information and training elements necessary for the implementation of the group's projects.

The objectives of the partnership are based on a network which takes place at several levels:

1 The initial network or heart of the project.
2 The district network.
3 The network in the conurbation of Rouen
4 The inter-project health network (RISS).
5 The international network.

1 The initial network or heart of the project

At this level, the objective is to work alongside the group so that it can enable *l'ause Bien Être* to mature according to the objectives it has set itself:

(a) Organise a permanent meeting place for women and men in need of recreation, to be less isolated and to share their problems and the search for solutions.
(b) Create projects around health and well-being, for example, personal image, relaxation and anti-stress techniques, dispensary for adults, support and self-help collective for parents of disabled children.
(c) Create specific workshops, for example, form-filling, gathering and distribution of information.

They have begun to do things together; three families have organised a holiday in VVF (Village Vacances Famille), and there have been common ventures and joint excursions (through RISS) to Paris and Lyon. As one member said:

In our group now, we can ask for help and accept it. In fact we are beginning to help each other, to talk about difficult problems and we realise that this means that we can bear them better and look for the solutions together.

2   The district network

At this level the objective is to find the necessary resources locally for the consolidation of the project and its recognition both in the district and in the town. It exists also to ensure that a diversity of groups meet up with each other in order to build a whole. Contact is being made with other associations or groups in the area. Links are being forged and people are being drawn closer together. Projects in common are being constructed and it could even go as far as putting together an association of local inhabitants made up of a range of groups.

3   The Rouen conurbation network

At this level, the objective is to open up the group, *Pause Bien Être*, to other experiences in the Rouennaise conurbation. A training development project meeting is set up in the area of Rouen on the theme of 'Bien dans sa vie, bien dans sa ville' (Content with life, content in your town). Three or four groups of local residents accompanied by social development workers are getting organised. A number of partners (formal organisations) support the project ethos:

> Development-training is based upon current experiences in the Rouen conurbation and allows the inhabitants and professionals to consolidate their action or to achieve projects which have made a step towards promoting health and social development. It will be a resource to be put at their disposal.
>
> (MDSL Practice Report)

Through the sharing of experiences already gained or about to be, the local residents should be able, working alongside social development and health professionals, to strengthen or confirm their role as parents. As well as being able to put forward their collective reaction, they can also work in depth on such themes as the law, authority, education of children and adolescents. In other respects, through work in the neighbourhood and the environment, residents' active role in the politics of the town will be constructed and defined with all the partners involved. The integration of the project *Pause Bien Être* into the growing network and organised in/around the conurbation should allow for a closer exchange of experiences.

4   The inter-project health network

At this level, the objective is to make the network RISS (Réseau InterSite Santé) a 'crucible' which will give the opportunity (through meeting residents of other areas and groups) of building together a resource centre, a place where exchange and the challenge of ideas allow local projects to be built.

Three projects are being networked at present in a national programme organised by the women inhabitants of Rouen, of Lyon and in Denain. The programme offers them the opportunity of sharing their experiences, of getting out and about, reaching a better understanding of their own lives by seeing what happens in other towns and how things might be changed at home.

For example, after a visit to Lyon, one woman from Rouen, seeing the 'miserable houses which you don't see anymore where we live' was to come to terms with the acute pain she had suffered and suppressed when, at 4 years old, she was evacuated with her family from Rouen to the suburbs. Becoming an active participant in her area and her town was born out of a sudden shedding of tears hundreds of kilometres away.

5   The international network

The networking of residents and professionals has grown into a community experience led by social psychologists with the residents in Rosario (Argentina). Residents from Rouen have been networking with residents from Rosario for the past three years. Saul Fuks, director of the Centre d'Aide à la Communauté, comes over from Argentina once a year to work as a consultant with residents and professionals. The more often that the women from Rouen made visits to Paris, Lyon or Bagneux and beyond, the more interested they have become in their own district. Think globally, act locally is the basis of all local social development action.

ACTION–TRAINING–RESEARCH – TRAINING DEVELOPMENT

Action–training–research is a permanent process of study, thought and the transformation of reality which calls for the participation in real and active terms of the people. Participation of the residents is not an alibi, a justification for professional action. It is a community exercise and

> is defined essentially as an exercise working alongside one or many activists in order to develop their capacity for analysis, to problem-solve, and to work out and realise their own projects. . . . The expert or the technician establishes a relationship of co-operation with the actors, contributes to the reinforcing of those capabilities of the actors, but is not a substitute for them.
>
> (Le Boterf and Lessard 1988)

Intervention hinges on three things – action, training and research – which interact on a permanent basis, the action being the essential element and objective of the process.

Action because the local participants have to solve real problems, take decisions, get projects under way, take the initiative.

Training because the process is conceived as being used in a teaching situation where the trainer 'accompanies the actors in their journey'. People as resources are identified, consulted or solicited for participation in support groups which can be either on a one-off or permanent basis.

Research which will allow the residents better to understand problems and situations in which they wish to intervene with the help of intermediaries. Collaborative research can also be put in place within the same framework. The professional works in tandem with the project, a helper who puts her knowledge and skills at the service of the shared activity of the group.

Development training rests on the assumption that each territory has under-exploited 'resources' which are latent or lying fallow and waiting to be discovered: physical resources, know-how, initiative and energy. The idea is that the training process can mobilise the locality. Development training should never be predetermined in the form of a fixed curriculum, but should be constructed according to the needs and demands of the local people and sustained by local bodies.

This kind of training is put together with the help of everybody concerned, from the promoters of the training and the institutions that support it to the participants who must play the main roles in the projects. The objective is the action to be carried out, and theoretical elements are included at the request of the participants in response to their questions or as research tools. Development training draws from the knowledge of trainees in order to give them the necessary tools to achieve their projects. It is offered to them as a resource. It is above all interactive and is enhanced each time that know-how is exchanged between participants.

Development training is built for and with the participants. It is conceived as alternating permanently between theory and practice. It is managed by a trainer who will run the scheme from beginning to end. She is there to work alongside the programme, build a training scheme with all the partners, and more specifically to sit in on the sessions with the participants themselves. She chooses her collaborators and answers for them.

Case study 2 – Canteloup

Development training as a tool of social development

In 1990 AIDE (Agence Intercommunale pour le Développement de l'Emploi – a training development agency) and CCAS (Centre Communal d'Action Sociale – local welfare services run by the commune) met and began a training project where the aim was to link the problem of child-minding in the town with a back to work programme for a number of women on the books of AIDE. They wanted to look after children as paid work. To do this, the women had to have access to approved nursery assistant status. A training was obviously necessary ('if we wanted a good standard of child minding') in order for the women to have access to a professional status.

In September 1991, MDSL-Formation was approached by AIDE to take on this training. They seized the opportunity to train the women and enable them to think about their role as women, as mothers and as future professionals in early childhood. The project was financed by the local authority, in partnership with a number of formal organisations. A steering committee was formed, made up of professionals from Canteloup (who had taken part in the recruitment of the trainees) as well as representatives from the administrative and departmental and regional medical authorities. The committee followed the project through from beginning to end.

Eventually, fourteen women between the ages of 25 and 45 with fifty-two children between them (average number of children per woman 3.8) took part. Their countries of origin included Morocco, Algeria and France. Only one of the women had never been to school. There was little formal academic achievement. The group elected two delegates who have regularly attended steering committee meetings.

The essential task was to make the women aware that they had the knowledge and the know-how while valuing their practical skills as mothers, and above all permitting them to establish links outside the area to compare the skills they acquired with other professionals. The content of the training is continually reworked in tandem with the concerns of the women. Teaching was interactive, allowing time for exchanges, to dynamise the group, to involve it and to allow its participation. The training timetable was essentially dictated by the family constraints of the women.

The co-ordination of the action was undertaken by a training officer with a nursing background, trained in the communitarian approach. She was supported by an MDSL-Formation worker who supported and worked alongside her. In order to enrich the training and widen the women's field of acquaintances, other helpers were invited to participate in the training.

The training for these women from Canteloup was 'an adventure'. This adventure became a project called *O comme trois pommes* (a name, a home, a dream – created together). The women say that they have acquired a certain self-affirmation, a greater understanding of identity, a shared knowledge of other communities in Canteloup:

> one of the auxiliaries/helpers told me that she could no longer accept her husband's disparaging remarks about 'magrébins' [people of North African origin] since knowing me.
>
> (*O comme trois pommes* participant)

They learned to establish a new relationship with the professionals in the town and to gain access to information. Other achievements include an awareness of the complexity involved in running a family and a job, an awareness of the responsibilities and the educational aspects involved in their roles as mothers and as future professionals and, for some, an improvement in their French – a passport to social and professional involvement.

Before and during the training, partnership work was widely de-veloped. It encouraged the establishment of an active network and activated a joint research initiative. All the professionals and the trainees were mobilised to work towards the future of the child in the city, no longer just in terms of ways/methods of child minding but also in terms of prevention and well-being. In spite of its limitations, access to nursery assistant training seems totally relevant to MDSL in order to reinforce the role of adults in the districts, to mobilise them, conferring respons-ibilities and validating their know-how, by recognising their gifts and developing their role in the network of institutions frequented by children.

There were limitations to the exercise beyond the short term. Not all of the institutions agreed with the initiative. Should MDSL-Formation accept such collaboration? It was clear that the synergy needed for the wider application of social development work tentatively put into action with the women's group was lacking. Yet, do we now abandon the work with the men and women from a district when they have responded with so much pleasure and enthusiasm from the outset? Development requires patience, time and commitment. One day perhaps these women -so aware during the training evaluation of the role they could play – might seize another opportunity to put to good use that which they began.

On the last day of the training session we talked to them about the conception and the vulnerability of all birth, of the time necessary for a child, like a project, to reach maturity. The project *O comme trois pommes* was compared to an egg. The last meeting was serious – after the couscous and the celebrations. If we were hoping that the next stage would follow on soon, they knew otherwise, that it would take time and they said so . . . wisely.

COLLABORATIVE RESEARCH

Collaborative research forms a special part in collective training for groups. It is a research method where, through their involvement in the research programme, the residents analyse their own situation and its problems, setting out guidelines which enable them to go from a common and fragmentary knowledge of social reality to a critical and plural knowledge of that same social reality. This research work helps them to resolve the problems identified, drawing from local resources. They can also become involved in the social development dynamic and play a part in the control of their social, family and personal lives.

The objectives fall into two categories; training and action. It allows for an awareness on the part of those surveyed of their problems and their determining factors. By objectifying problems, proposals can be drawn up by the groups involved in the research so that actions can be taken, capable of resolving the problems and drawing on local resources. Collaborative research must be adapted to the particular conditions of the local situation. However, the theoretical frame of reference of any joint/social survey involves four phases dictated by a time limit plus the feedback of those research findings. It is at this stage that the shared and communitarian dynamic can be amplified through discussion, criticism and questioning of the research and the action by the members of the community. The shared process of action–training–research is a dynamic, recursive and non-linear process. There are four possible phases of a joint survey:

- structure and methods realised conjointly by the promoters of the research and the representatives of the local participants;
- preliminary and provisional study of the area and the population concerned;
- critical analysis of the problems considered by the population to be a priority and which its members wish to study and resolve;
- programming and establishment of a plan of action for the resolution of those problems.

Case study 3 – Collaborative research as a tool of social development: developing integration in Rouen

First of all eleven and then fifteen residents of a district of Rouen, who wanted to change and improve their quality of life, came together in a group in order to produce a social development project. The preparation work of the survey was conducted once a week from May to July increasing during August. Several members of MDSL-Formation took part and a doctor, a sociologist, the director of MDSL, a local councillor and an urban architect helped with the work of developing the survey questionnaire especially about housing, environment and play areas. The facilitators of the group were local-patch social workers. They were not however relieved of their usual workload, not even slightly.

First of all, the group stuck to clarifying and redefining its expectations where the survey was concerned. The thoughts most representative of the group included:

- get closer to people;
- speak to other people;
- get out of the ghetto more;
- change mentalities;
- change one's own way of looking at problems;
- find a better way of life/live better.

Fears and potential obstacles were also defined; for example, fear of being ignored and being resigned to a fear of a number of aggressive people. The members of the group were particularly aware of the difficulty of going to meet other residents whom they did not know. A second job was that of redefinition, aimed at understanding the knowledge of the technical terms frequently employed by professionals but little used by the residents; for example, survey, collaborative/action research, multiple factors, networking, social development, auto-biography. A third task was to locate and map primary networks by/of members of the group in the area, in order to pinpoint the people who would be most easily contactable and easily mobilised by the group.

We then restructured the research and the work in progress in a more global approach to social development in order to clarify the positions and the roles of each participant in the project. This job allowed the members of the group to prepare more easily for the meetings with professionals or elected members of the municipality. A colleague brought along and shared with the group some tools of communication and worked at the development of an 'information letter' on activities and projects for the district which the group then distributed to 800 homes in the district.

This distribution was done in such a way that it was not merely a transfer of information but was used as a first contact to gauge the interest of the residents in the work of the group and also as a starter to engage people around the survey. Seven hundred and forty-nine contacts were recorded and thirty-eight reply coupons were analysed with the social workers.

From this period came the redefinition of the aims of the survey, which were to:

• have ideas and opinions;
• take part with other residents in a development programme in the district;
• produce concrete things;
• discover 'know how';
• inform others, inform oneself.

Major themes to be discussed with the other residents corresponded to the major preoccupations of the group: play areas, youth, housing, work, unemployment, career/job, life in the area, the environment, safety, health. After clarifying the themes, questions were formulated using three criteria. What information do we want to obtain? Why is it necessary? What do we want to show using this information?

It is to this long and arduous job that most of the month of August 1993 was devoted in order to carry out the survey at the beginning of September. A letter with the results of the survey was drafted. Distributing a newsletter requires communications techniques which had to be acquired. An interviewer's guide was drawn up to make the job easier. A workshop with the Theatre of the Oppressed (Boal 1992) made it possible to prepare for meeting other residents. The final act of preparation for the survey was to have a run through of the questionnaire with twenty or so people as a test of its quality. The analysis of the questionnaires circulated, the mistakes made and the difficulties encountered allowed for the redefinition of the way in which the questionnaire was administered.

Following this test, the questionnaire was shortened and some of the questions modified, which resulted in the definitive version comprising 226 questions. Table 10.1 shows the percentage of questions by theme.

Table 10.1 Percentage of questions by theme

Themes	Number of Questions	%
General	15	6.64
Play Areas	45	19.91
Youth	12	5.31
Housing	32	14.16
Work/unemployment/career	49	21.68
Life in the district	27	11.95
Environment	8	3.54
Security/safety	9	3.98
Health	29	12.83
Total	226	100

It was decided after several meetings running in June 1993 that the theme of play areas for children would be treated as a priority. Information was received from the mayor's office to the effect that a sum of money had been allotted for the improvement of open spaces of the area because the area used by the children for play space was now dilapidated.

Bearing in mind the wishes and capabilities of the group it was decided to practise what was called a 'cooptation affective' ('engage your friends!'). The ties of friendship and solidarity which unified them made it easier for them to complete the task. This approach was of course less representative and a more risky sample. But it is quite sufficient in such a context. What is lost in representation is gained in efficiency.

The survey itself was then able to be started and 149 people were interviewed between 30 August and 14 September 1993. All were residents of the district of Rouen. The sample was mainly made up of women (69.1 per cent compared to 54 per cent in the Census).

The part of the research concerning play areas was made available to the residents and key professionals in the district during a 'theatre-forum' with the Theatre of the Oppressed at the social centre in the area. To prepare for the dissemination the results were analysed by the residents in the group, social workers and training officers from MDSL-Formation.

Posters were made. Written commentaries accompanied the posters and verbal explanations were given to the participants at the forum. These posters allowed the other residents to see that the replies they had given during the survey were taken into consideration and were useful to the establishment of a play-space project. The other participants at the forum were able to appreciate all the work produced. At the end of the forum, ten adults and children enrolled as helpers in the play-space project.

During a day out at the premises of MDSL-Formation given over to the evaluation of the work of the enquiry, the residents of the group were able to see the results of their research. The computer presentation attracted a lively interest. The residents said that they were not able to measure the importance of their own work. However, later each woman made an evaluation of her own initiative during the course of the survey. The residents were very much aware of the importance of interviewing their friends and neighbours. The task was far easier than they had thought, but as one resident described her experience:

I turned up at my friends' homes, was made very welcome but when it came to other people, doors were closed.

The women observed that the fact of being in a group where you expressed yourself in many languages had advantages when it came to communicating with different ethnic groups. For example:

Some people did not speak French. I translated into Woloff and after that Marie-Thérèse was able to communicate – it was cool!

The residents felt validated by the local populace from whom they received encouragement, sympathy and support. Moreover, they learnt much about their district and themselves. We should note that collaborative research is a means of understanding, analysing the social environment and proposing actions to solve real problems. This only has a value if the residents themselves own the production of it. The knowledge produced during this exercise is and will remain the basis of their project development. We have seen how, having learnt that the local council envisaged an improvement in the play spaces in the area, the group had decided to seize the opportunity to produce one of the priorities of the social survey. The local council wanted to install the play equipment fast, but the group suggested that they await the results of the survey on play spaces. The council accepted the suggestion. Later, the group members negotiated to develop a play-space building project with the technical services of the town.

To allow the group to acquire the necessary tools to make the

214 Marie-Renée Bourget-Daitch & Chris Warren

play-area building happen (for example, reading of the plans of the site and the district, choice of site for the play space, study of the equipment and urban building), technical training was provided by a colleague. It was carried out in the district social centre, and beyond; for example, the Honoré de Balzac Primary School where they were able to see a model produced by the students which showed the building of the play area on an adjacent plot, Honoré de Balzac Nursery School where the children had made drawings of their ideal play areas, and in Paris where they visited the St Ambroise Square, the Belleville Gardens, and the Buttes-Chaumont Park.

The residents began to realise that they could be involved and be 'go-betweens' for the partnership organisations at municipal level in particular. The play-space project was both a means and an end. An end because it was seeking an objective which was to 'have a place where our kids can play' – but it was also a means because through this project the residents were involved in the life of their district, as citizens. The council decided on outside play spaces and adopted the residents' project. The council architect used most of the plan put forward by the group.

VIDEO SURVEY: A SOCIAL SURVEY OF A PARTICULAR KIND

A case study – the video as a tool of social development: *Nous . . . St Martin* – Limeil-Bravannes

MDSL-Formation established an action–training–research project as part of the Développement Social des Quartiers (DSQ) – a community development initiative in Limeil-Brevannes, based on a theme of 'health and well-being'.

MDSL worked with residents in the area, people under contract with the workshop *Nous . . . St Martin*, the local organisation responsible for establishing the DSQ development at local level, along with development staff. The process was as follows:

Preparatory phase April to September

For MDSL-Formation, the start of the action in an area is established from a process, a dynamic and not from a procedure with rigid rules. MDSL-Formation had been approached earlier by a local group, at which time the residents had already undergone two or three difficult phases with the feeling in some quarters that they had been 'abandoned'.

MDSL-Formation took part in re-engaging the residents in working alongside a masters student of social development at the University of Villetaneuse. After the first meeting with this group of twenty or so people, MDSL-Formation established two training days on the theme:

> Knowledge of the district, of its habitat, of its inhabitants, of it environment, of its place in the town and in the wider community. How do we live, get out and progress? What are the potentialities, its weaknesses, its dynamics?

To help the group in the job of deciphering the day to day reality, Jean-Loup Herbert, (anthropologist and lecturer at the school of architecture in Saint Etienne) was approached. A wander about the district allowed the group to see the advantages, the problems and the decline, as well as the reason for hope of renewal. This phase for us proved to be essential. We could not in fact turn up without being invited and welcomed by those who live in the area. Philippe Macquet, director of the Maison Régionale de Promotion de la Santé du Nord Pas-de-Calais, says about this first phase:

> When I arrive at people's homes, I ring the bell, wipe my feet on the mat, I have a bunch of flowers in my hand and I wait for them to invite me in. Without these preliminary gestures you risk being an intruder in a district.

Awareness phase and training of the participants. From September to November: working alongside residents

Our team worked as much with the operational team as with the members of the group who little by little took on the name of pilot group in order to put the survey work properly in place. The survey should be thought of as a tool/skill, a means to serve the population and not as an end in itself. This was the concern of the local councillor, responsible for the Développement Social des Quartiers, and president of the association *Nous . . . Saint Martin.*

Some people thought that once recruited to the survey they had to wait for orders and the tools (questionnaire and specific training) would be given to them to carry out the project. It did nothing for their sense of security to hear from MDSL-Formation that it was they the residents who should know what information they wanted to find out about their district and that they had to go out to meet the other residents to find out what they needed to do to develop the research. At the end of October, awareness that this was their business and theirs alone became evident, and they chose the annual festival as the best moment to go out to meet the other residents. The investigation took the form of a video in the street.

Establishing the action/phase. Production of communication skills and production of knowledge with deconstruction and reconstruction of local realities.

The preparatory work for the video enquiry considered four questions:

• What do you think of the area?
• What do you think of the youth/adults relationship?
• What is your main preoccupation?
• Do you have a passion to share?

The street video took place in November during the festival. Fifty or so people were interviewed of both sexes and of all ages. A professional video maker, Isabelle Mammoliti, lent her technical support to this stage. The video was finished in the following March, entirely produced by a small group of residents who gained skills at different stages of the development of the product. The film lasted about ten minutes, and was a tool capable of inspiring meetings with other residents in the area and inviting them to take part in a dialogue. The producers were careful to show in the film everybody they had interviewed in the district – even if their opinion was not selected. In this sense the film was like a family album of the district and was a starting point for meetings. The video title was 'Saint Martin, c'est nous!'

At the same time as we developed the synopsis, we worked on the distribution phase and the showing of the film. The work was formalised by a meeting of those in the network. The main idea was to be able to reach as many people as possible at varying dates and projection times, which required no small investment in time and availability. During April and May 1994, viewing sessions took place for the 'Saint Martin, c'est nous!' video with children, parents and youth groups plus nine elected representatives from the town council, including the mayor. The reactions were positive each time. A policy grew little by little to enlarge the vision of the residents of the area and hence the awareness of the possibilities of change they could initiate so that life could improve and a sense of well-being be reborn. When MDSL-Formation stopped the first phase of its work, an analysis of the 'St Martin, c'est nous!' video sessions showed that there were two major concerns: education of children (6 to 12 year-olds in particular), and the general needs of young people in the area.

We concluded that the priority was to establish open training for all parents and adults concerned with this age group. This training could be the space where, while increasing residents' knowledge and skill towards children, parents and adults, medical, social and community workers could build together an original policy of prevention. The work began in the group called *Accueil des Enfants*, which would offer the framework in which this training action could be constructed. The interest of the young in the district – their wish to see their image improve becoming more and more obvious – could be reinforced by giving them the opportunity of a 'creativity workshop on knowing the area', having as objectives:

• learn to have a stake in the district, in the town, in the pattern of places, partnerships and institutions, jurisdiction (procedures and rules);
• learn to express and formalise the representation of the town and of the district;
• learn to do a project together: first by planning and secondly by putting it into effect.

The work of the MDSL-Formation with *Nous . . . Saint Martin* was originally fixed at six months. In reality, because of administrative delays and then because of the pace of the residents, it took place over a period of over eighteen months with a six-month intensive phase. During this period the MDSL-Formation, along with other initiatives, lost its mandate from the town and work ceased. Nevertheless, the video inquiry goes well. It proves that residents can meet each other, get to know each other, rediscover each other, and that the making and building of things together are in themselves important. In the evaluation session of their work with the pilot group which was the last session of work in common:

> The group in its entirety declared itself to be very satisfied with the work achieved. In fact, in the legitimate satisfaction of having brought to term a long and difficult task, came the pleasure in producing a product of quality which was remarked upon by all its viewers. . . . These sessions gave to the group members a . . . positive image of their actions.

CONCLUSION

We have described the work of MDSL-Formation, a French social development agency with a focus on working alongside local people in a process called action–training–development. We want to emphasise in our conclusion that the values and techniques of social development described above are not unique but that they are being applied now, that they are applied to the world of children and families, and they are being reproduced and shared widely. Moreover, we should like to underline three of the messages from this account of MDSL-Formation's action: (a) the special role of the development team in local partnership; (b) its ability to engage expertise from people with shared values; (c) the emphasis on community networking and the principle of 'act local, think global'.

NOTE

This chapter is based on a practice report by MDSL-Formation entitled 'Pour une maîtrise et une appropriation par les habitants de leur vie, de leur santé, et de leur environnement', written by M.-R. Bourget-Daitch and B. Pissaro (in collaboration with the Laboratoire de Santé Public – Faculté Saint Antoine, Université Pierre et Marie Curie – Paris, and l'Association FIPE Santé-DOC).

REFERENCES

Boal, A. (1992) *Games for Actors and Non-Actors*, London, Routledge.
Freire, P. (1972) *Pedagogy of the Oppressed*, Harmondsworth, Penguin.
Le Boterf, G. and Lessard, P. (1988) *L'Ingénerie des Projets de Développement – Gestion Participative et Développement Institutionel*, Paris, Editions Païdeia.
MDSL (1995) Le Mouvement pour un Développement Social Local-Formation: 52 rue du Four, 75006 Paris. Tel. (1) 45 44 65 10.
Rosnay, J. de (1984) *Les Chemins de la Vie*, Paris, Seuil.
Speck, R.V. and Attneave, C. L. (1973) *Family Networks*, New York, Vintage.

Index

The following abbreviations have been used in the index:

FGCs Family Group Conferences
SC Save the Children